In Pursuit of Healing

In Pursuit of Healing

❖

Breaking the Chains That Prevent Healing

Carl Townsend

iUniverse, Inc.
New York Lincoln Shanghai

In Pursuit of Healing
Breaking the Chains That Prevent Healing

iUniverse, Inc.

For information address:
iUniverse, Inc.
2021 Pine Lake Road, Suite 100
Lincoln, NE 68512
www.iuniverse.com

Cover Design by Robilyn Robbins

ISBN: 0-595-29308-5 (pbk)
ISBN: 0-595-65986-1 (cloth)

Printed in the United States of America

Contents

Acknowledgements

Thanks to my editors. Thanks to Wayne McCroskey, who with his wife Sandy did a perfectionist job on the original manuscript. Thanks to Toni Anderson, who edited with an engaging dialog which I wish could have been put beside the text here. You will find a few of her questions in the chapter dialog areas. Any errors that remain are my own—they did a great job.

Thanks to Robilyn Robbins for the cover design. The cover is based on a banner Robilyn designed for East Hills Foursquare Church in Gresham, Oregon.

Thanks to my pastor, Kevin Carlisle, for his dialog on the issues and support. Some of his wonderful sermon stories slipped in here and there.

And a special thanks to Jesus of Nazareth, the real author of my faith and this book.

Introduction

I am thanking you, God, from a full heart,
I'm writing the book on your wonders.
I'm whistling, laughing, and jumping for joy;
I'm singing your song, High God.

—Ps. 9:1–2 *The Message*

During the three years from 1989 to 1992, I experienced two incredibly deep spiritual journeys. First, in June of 1989 I was suddenly paralyzed by a virus in Zermatt, Switzerland and was told by the doctors I would never walk again. I walked again over a year later, unassisted. Just as I started walking again (1991), my wife started a battle with leukemia, and even with a bone marrow transplant I lost her a little over a year later.

In both of these, I walked through some very deep waters. With the first, I really believed if I had enough faith I could walk again. I read the Acts 3 story of the lame man several times every day until I walked again. I had to know how that lame man in the Bible walked. Then, when my wife had leukemia, we bought the same vision—only she didn't get well. I had been praying for her. Friends had been praying for her. The family had been praying for her. The church had been praying for her. People around the world prayed for her. Then we lost her. She was one of the greatest gifts God had ever given me. It's not fair for someone to give you a gift and then take it back. God wasn't even being ethical, in my mind. God sets the game and the rules, however. Not us. What happened? Was my faith lacking? Did I need more faith? I could see in the Bible where Jesus was constantly chiding his disciples for their lack of faith. Was I at the same place? What a guilt trip!

IDENTIFYING THE PROBLEM

I did realize, however, that the problem was one of prayer. I didn't know enough about prayer. There was really no one to blame but myself. I would need to travel to the best of prayer conferences and sit at the feet of the best pray-ers in the world to learn some things about prayer. What I didn't realize was that now that I had this insight from God, the Enemy was going to launch his best attack yet. The Enemy *knew* prayer worked.

THE NEXT ATTACK

The first prayer conference I attended was in 1993, and it was a doozy. It was on the east side of Seattle, and I rode up from Portland with a well-known prayer and deliverance minister, Tom White. That night as I registered at the conference motel, I suddenly became sick, violently throwing up. Racing through the crowd of distinguished prayer warriors in the lobby, I was trying to find the rest room in a strange motel. Later, as I reached my room (I was rooming with Tom), I staggered to my bed as Tom saw the carnage.

"Carl," you look like you're going to die."

"I feel like it, too." I replied.

"Ever had this before?"

"No, never."

That night I tossed and turned. There was no fever, no diarrhea. Just a wrestling with my pillow that continued all night.

The next morning I lay there in bed, exhausted but recovering.

"How are you doing?" Tom asked.

"Better. A little weak, but the breakfast should fix that. Tom, can you help me?"

"Nope." he replied.

"I'm serious."

Then Tom sat up on the side of his bed and read off a litany of the warfare battles I was currently involved in.

"Nope," he said, "I can't help you."

I was fine as the conference continued, although one of the conference intercessors did tap me on the shoulder that day asking if I needed prayer. I took him up on that.

While coming home with Tom, he gave me some specific prophecies. They all came true within two months.

After I got home I called my doctor.

"How long," I said, "after exposure to tainted food does it take for a stomach 'flu' to attack?"

"About four or five hours," he said.

"I prayed and fasted that day going into the conference. I hadn't eaten anything."

"It wasn't a virus or bacteria." he said. "You need to up your prayer level. I have a small group that can take you if you need it." My doctor knew I was in danger. He knew my history and commitment.

"Thanks. I'm in a small group now."

I continued processing the events with other mentors. It soon became apparent what was happening. One mentor pointed out to me that the conference was within only a few miles of the transplant center where my wife had gotten her bone marrow transplant and then later died. Furthermore, I noticed then that each time I went to Seattle after that I would get hit with a similar, but less virulent, form of attack. To put it bluntly from the information in Daniel, I didn't know enough about the territorial guy over that city (see Daniel 10). My pastor at the time discerned this and launched a prayer targeted at this guy. The problem was resolved. Several times since then I have gone to conferences (two of them were prayer conferences in the same city) and found them to be wonderful experiences of praise and celebration.

Prayer leaders who lead these conferences have also learned more about prayer. For example, using lots of praise music really gets the Enemy ticked off. Today these prayer conferences I go to always bring in a very strong worship leader or group, and the praise music is used at the beginning of every session.

During the next few years I went to conference after conference on prayer. I sat at the feet of Dean Sherman, Dick Eastman, George Otis, Jr., Francis Frangipane, Rolland Smith, Tom White, Peter Wagner, Bob Becket, Chuck Kraft, Alistar Petrie, Dutch Sheets, Victor Lorenzo, Sondra Hampe, John Dawson, Ed Silvoso, Graham Cooke, Jack Dennison, Peter Bachelder, Bob Waymire, and more to listen to their teaching. Much of this book contains teachings distilled from these.

Two key questions I asked of God as I started my search:

1. Why didn't Sandy get well? (This is the wrong questions to ask, I learned later. There is, however, a right question.)

2. Why was this list of prayer warriors almost all men?

WHERE WE WILL GO

The title of this book seems to indicate we do something to initiate the healing. We do, but it's probably not what you think. There are no "steps to healing." Jesus always seemed to do it different each time. Was there anything in common with all the healings? (Yes.)

In this book we will look at some of these issues. In particular, we will look at some of the healings Jesus did. I say this with caution because remember there is really no formula for healing. Sometimes faith of the healed preceded healing; sometimes the healing preceded their faith. Always, however, the faith of Jesus preceded the healing. Sometimes Jesus didn't seem to give a dingy whether the hurting person had enough faith or not. Then at Nazareth the Bible makes it plain Jesus couldn't do his healing there "because of their unbelief." What's with this, anyway?

You may be reading this book because you need healing yourself. You are not alone. We are all wounded. Now let's continue and look at some of the real issues in healing.

THE ECHO

When authoring this book, certain phrases and scriptures came up again and again. Toward the end I began to tackle the task of eliminating this duplication of the verses. It seemed, however, the Lord begged me not to do this. What he told me is that when you read it the first time you won't believe it. When you read it the second time you won't believe it. By the time you get to the end of the book, maybe there is enough faith to take a tiny step. That is what I'm praying for you. That is all it takes to move mountains.

> *"All Jesus did that day was tell stories—a long storytelling afternoon.*
> *His storytelling fulfilled the prophecy:*
> *'I will open my mouth and tell stories;*
> *I will bring out into the open*
> *things hidden since the world's first day.'"*
> —Matt. 13: 34–35 *The Message*

> *"One of our crises is that Christianity has presented itself as a system of belief instead of a story. Christ did not die for a belief or an idea. Christ died for you."*

1

The Great Myth

"The hands of the king are the hands of a healer. And so shall the rightful king be known."

—Ioreth, in *The Lord of the Rings: The Return of the King*

I love chocolate-covered cake donuts. When I was a kid, my dad would sometimes bring a box of them home and we would devour them. Dad was quite a teaser, and one day he cautioned me.

"Carl, be very careful you don't eat the hole in the donut. The hole in the donut is poisonous, and if you get into that you might get sick or even die."

After that, I tried to be careful. It wasn't too long, however, before I got sick after eating one of those donuts. I was very sure I had accidentally gotten into the hole of the donut. Of course, it wasn't caused by the donut hole, but no one could convince me it wasn't. For a long time after that, whenever I ate a donut I was very careful to leave a little ring of donut right around the hole.

Now what my father told me was a myth.[1] It had absolutely no truth at all. A lie. Yet I not only believed it, but I also acted on it as if it were true. There was a lot of anxiety and a wonderful piece of the donut left every time I ate one because I was living in a small story. My unbelief (or rather belief in what was not true) kept me from embracing the larger story.

Isn't that much like our spiritual journey? In our growing up we may have heard many stories about the Christian faith; but the faith's basic nature is so radical, so unbelievable, and so incredible that we

1

never really rest in it and act into it with total abandon. We stay in our small story.

THE PARABLE OF THE RIVER

I think God gets his kicks by doing extraordinary things that look very wild to us. You don't have to read very far in the Bible to see this. Noah builds this weird boat and then fills it up with all kinds of animals. He tells Abraham to kill his first-born son of promise, then stays Abraham's hand as he is about to sacrifice this only son. With God's help Moses leads a nation through a parted sea. He feeds the Israelites as they travel through a wilderness. David kills a giant with a slingshot. There is the fiery furnace, the repentance of an entire city (Nineveh). God tells a prophet to bury his underpants, and then dig them up later. God tells another prophet to marry a harlot. A Jewish virgin lady marries a heathen Gentile king to save her nation. Peter is released from prison by an angel. Paul and Silas (as they are singing praise music) are released from prison in the middle of the night by an earthquake. The Apostle Paul breaks bread to eat on a ship in the middle of a storm. God still does weird things like this. He hasn't changed.

As a contemporary comparison, near my house the Tualatin River flows to the Willamette River. Sometimes in the morning I drive down Childs Road, following the Tualatin River, to a restaurant for breakfast. In 1996, however, the river flooded into the houses along the road and over the road. The road was a lake. This road along the river was closed. The houses on this road were all damaged by the flood. There were a lot of "For Sale" signs after the river receded and the houses repaired. Other people along the road, however, decided to stay. After all, the river only flooded once every hundred years.

A year later in 1997 the river flooded again, the road was closed again, and the houses repaired again. The real cause of the flooding was never dealt with. Upstream from the flooding the housing and business density had increased dramatically, and what had been rural land that could absorb the overflow was now hard with asphalt and cement and could not absorb the water. There was no longer enough drainage for the river as it wandered through the town of Tualatin and down to the Willamette River, eventually to the Columbia. The dams and locks were simply not enough to contain it. And they still aren't.

God's actions in our world are much like this river. It really doesn't matter much what we believe or do to stop his advance today. Like the wild river, he continues to flow through our lives, cities, and homes, bringing healing and joy where the heart is hungry and thirsty. We may carry our myths and small stories; but the coming of the Kingdom is not limited by our small stories. God can still heal, raise people from the dead, enable the lame to walk, and bring Good News to the poor. For those captive, hungry, and who have eyes to see and ears to hear, God will make himself known. I've seen and heard all of this.

WHY ARE WE HERE?

Of all the creations of God, Man is the only thing that was created with a hunger, desire, and thirst for something beyond himself (or herself). *Unlike any other being, Man carries a deep yearning for something long lost. There is a passionate sense of adventure to discover what this is that was lost.*

As Morpheus says in *The Matrix*:

> *"What you know you can't explain, but you feel it. You've felt it your entire life, that there's something wrong with the world. You don't know what it is, but it's there, like a splinter in your mind, driving you mad."*

God created Man for intimacy with him, and that relationship was lost with the Fall in the Garden of Eden. From that time on, Man has tried to get back to that place, a place of wellness and intimacy with God. God wants us well, or healed. We were created to glorify him.

The Enemy got a foothold in the Garden, but God provided a way out and eventual healing with his Son, Jesus.

This Garden is not so much a geographic place as a place of unity with our Creator. It is a place of wellness and healing that is achieved from this intimacy. It is a place for which Man was created in the first place. It is a place where we are healed. We desire healing; God desires us to be healed.

Man tries to reach this Garden on his own. In Genesis we see him building a Tower of Babel to reach this place. It hasn't been that many centuries since Man left Europe to find the New World. A place with a Fountain of Youth and Cities of Gold. Then the earlier pioneers left their comfortable lives on the east coast to move west. The early pioneers to my city of Portland were looking for Eden. Now with our rockets into space we are at it again. People argue after space tragedies whether Man should go into space. It is not a choice, Man is called to space. This search is not something we choose. It is built in us. Animals don't have this hunger. It's a deep hunger, a desire for something beyond description that will give us the healing we desire and can only be found in our relationship to him, who created us in the first place.

In the same way, God is always there and acting in our life to capture our heart and bring us to him. Whether we believe it or not, he is there and acting. We may not like his agenda for us, but his purpose is always the same—to win our heart. He is always seeking to heal us, but with his agenda, not ours.

As I write this, if it is a sunny day I can look out my window and see Mt. Hood, a two-mile high mountain, soaring into the sky. Today it is cloudy. The mountain is not visible. Yet I still believe the mountain is there, even though I can't see it. Whether I believe in the mountain or not makes no difference to it being there. It is there. The same is true of God. Whether we believe in him or not, he still is acting in our life. He wants us well.

When a child sees his or her mother or father leave the room, that parent ceases to exist for the child. The child doesn't realize the parent is still there, only in another room. In the same way, we are all children of our Heavenly Father. When one of his children dies, we weep because from our perception they are no longer there. But they really are there, still acting in our lives. Hebrews 12:1 makes that plain.

> *"Therefore we also, since we are surrounded by so great a cloud of witnesses, let us lay aside every weight, and the sin which so easily ensnares us, and let us run with endurance the race that is set before us"*
>
> —Heb 12:1 NKJV

Notice they are not just above us or beside us they *surround* us. The word used in the Greek for "surround" is *perikeimai*, which means to encircle, enclose, or to be bound with. The Enemy can't get through.

And then again in Revelation:

> *"And the smoke of the incense, with **the prayers of the saints**, ascended before God from the angel's hand. Then the angel took the censer, filled it with fire from the altar, and threw it to the earth. And there were noises, thunderings, lightnings, and an earthquake."*
>
> —Rev 8:4–5 NKJV, emphasis added

God and those before us are still there, whether we believe and can accept that or not.

WHO IS THE HEALER?

In J. R. R. Tolkien's *Lord of the Rings: The Return of the King,* the saving of Middle Earth doesn't look promising. The city has been destroyed by the enemy and even the gates are torn down. Aragorn, who they expected to be the coming King, has left for the Paths of the Dead with his few followers, a place from which no human has ever returned alive. No one has heard from Frodo and his friend Sam (little halflings who are less than four feet tall) since they left for the enemy's dark territory to throw the ring in the volcano from which it was forged, saving Middle Earth. Denethor, the Steward of the City (there had been no King for a long time) had given up hope and committed suicide. Denethor also tried to kill his son, Faramir, who now lays near death in one of the Houses of Healing. Merry, one of our dear hobbits, lies near death in another of the Houses of Healing. Lady Eowyn, as well, lies dying in the Houses of Healing.

> *"...till at last the red sunset filled all the sky, and the light through the windows fell on the grey faces of the sick. Then it seemed to those who stood by that in the glow the faces flushed softly with health returning, but it was only a mockery of hope.*
>
> *Then an old wife, Ioreth, the eldest of the women who served in that house, looking on the fair face of Faramir, wept, for all the people loved him. And she said: 'Alas! if he should die. Would that there were kings in Gondor, as there were once upon a time, they say! For it is said in old lore:* **The hands of the king are the hands of a healer**. *And so the rightful king could ever be known.'*
>
> *And Gandalf, who stood by, said: 'Men may long remember your words, Ioreth! For there is hope in them.'"*
>
> —J. R. R. Tolkien, *The Lord of the Rings: The Return of the King*

I wept as I read this. Far too many times I have prayed for someone trying to bring healing to that person. In reality I wanted to be the hero. Finally, when I gave up, I released the healing to Jesus, the ultimate Healer and King. Within minutes the healing would be there.

As Tolkien's story continues, Ioreth is unaware that Aragorn *has* returned and camped at the bottom of the hill below the city with a massive army he has brought with him. Aragorn sends a messenger up to ask permission to enter the city. The gates are destroyed, but Aragorn still seeks permission. Aragorn then learns the Steward of the city is dead. Next, Aragorn sends the messenger to ask for permission from the next in line, only to be told the son lies near death in the Houses of Healing. It is then that Aragorn enters the city. He brings the desired healing to Faramir, Lady Eowyn, and Merry.

> *"Suddenly Faramir stirred, and he opened his eyes, and he looked on Aragon who bent over him; and a light of knowledge and love was kindled in his eyes, and he spoke, softly. 'My Lord, you called me. I come. What does the King command?' 'Walk no more in the shadows, but awake!' said Aragorn."*
>
> —J. R. R. Tolkien, *The Lord of the Rings: The Return of the King*

Finally, with the final destruction of the Ring in the volcano, Aragorn is crowned as King.

I could not help, as I read this, to wonder if Tolkien had ever traveled to St. Paul's cathedral in London and seen the famous painting that hangs there. The painting shows Christ at the door, knocking. But there is one strange thing about the door—there is no doorknob. The door can only be opened from the inside! As with Aragorn, here is the King, the healer, asking to come into your heart. Yet Jesus is not going to do it unless you invite him in for the healing. He's too much of a gentleman. And what will you give Jesus permission to do? Open the front door, but let some of those other rooms in your heart stay locked? Are you really going to open up everything?

DO YOU BELIEVE?

Jesus made it quite clear that the only path to salvation and healing was though him:

> *"Jesus said to him, 'I am the way, the truth, and the life. No one comes to the Father except through Me.'"*
>
> —John 14:6 NKJV

Do you believe these words of Jesus? He is the only path we have.

What happens if you believe? Can you really risk it? The biggest stronghold we face is often the stronghold of unbelief. Can you take that step?

> *"One of the reasons we don't see more miracles is because we don't expect them."*
>
> —Dutch Sheets

Jesus faced this same stronghold in the lives of his disciples; yet he had only a short time to train them and move them beyond that unbelief. One of these lessons is in Matthew 14:22–23, a course which Francis Frangipane refers to as Water Walking 101. You'd think if Jesus was going to teach them how to walk on the water, he would start on a small pond that was shallow on a nice day and work up to the big stuff. No, he has to start them on the Sea of Galilee in the middle of a storm.

Jesus had been having some quiet time with his Father up on the mountain after feeding the five thousand. The disciples got in a boat at the Sea of Galilee and pushed off. Now it's night, a storm comes up, and they are three or four miles from the coast. Jesus comes walking across the water to the boat in the darkness, seeming to them much as a ghost or apparition. The disciples are afraid.

Jesus calls out to them to not be afraid, but it is only Peter who is able to discern it is Jesus. (How do you think Peter discerned this?) Peter calls out to Jesus that if it is he, bid him to come to Jesus. Jesus' reply is simple, "Come." Peter gets out of the boat and begins walking to Jesus. I like the way Frangipane tells this.

> *"Peter never walked on the water. He walked on [in obedience to] the words of Jesus."*

We often criticize Peter because he begins to fall in the water after walking a short distance. The rest of the disciples, however, never got out of the boat. Are you willing to get out of the boat? What are you walking on?

Can you move beyond any binding you have from the Enemy and the culture about you?

Dialog

1. What myths about healing exist in your life? Why are they there?

2. What risks are you taking today to move beyond those myths? Are you willing to take them?

3. What forces prevent you from taking that risk?

4. How do you think Peter recognized the voice of Jesus? How do you?

5. What does this mean in your personal life: "The gates are gone, but the King still seeks permission"?

Notes

1. A *myth* is a story that has universal truth. It may be true, or it may not be true in fact, but does carry a universal truth. The creation story is true, but is also a myth. *Lord of the Rings* is a myth, but is not true in fact. Part of our problem today is the impoverishment of our myths; that is, we have few stories strong enough to carry us through the healing for which we cry. Watch where the stories in this book come from: the movies, the comic pages, and a magazine advertisement. Our video games can also carry strong myths (as the *Myst* game). Most of the stories Christ told where spoken from the Agricultural Paradigm of the day. He described the Kingdom to his followers through the use of stories that carried universal truths (myths). We need leaders today to give us new stories that

are strong enough today to give us the deep truths of the Kingdom and to the healing Jesus brings.

2

The Pursuit of Intimacy

"Some things have to be believed to be seen."

Prayer, intimacy, and healing are all related. Jesus spent most of his ministry life in an intimate relationship with the Father and either praying or healing. Everything was related. This means that if you expect healing or the ministry of healing others, you need to learn an awful lot about praying and building intimacy with God. To those that followed, he spoke in strange parables about the Kingdom.

THE STARTING POINT FOR INTIMACY

At my church we had been doing various prayer events, but we desired training in teaching people who had the calling to be part of a healing ministry on how to do effective prayer; that is, if they prayed for someone we could expect healing. As a starting point, we decided to get some video training from someone who was already living at this level as well as some help from another church that had leadership in this area.

Our pastor (and wife) then said before we could do this we needed to take two other courses. One of these was on how to build a deep, intimate, relationship with God. The second course was on how to listen to God. Without the intimacy and the ability to listen, you can't discern or hear what God's agenda is all about. Shortly after our church began the first course on building intimacy with God, I attended a prayer conference with Graham Cooke. His first session was on how to build intimacy with God. I was beginning to get the message.

Your task, then, as you begin to experience healing or to help another person experience healing, is to build this intimacy with God. What, exactly, does that mean?

A PARABLE ABOUT INTIMACY

If you have a good marriage, you probably already know a few things about intimacy. I grew up as an independent guy. I could go into my "lab" and do all kinds of scientific things and mom would shove sandwiches under the door to keep me going. Computers were predictable as long as I understood how they worked. People (particularly women) were not; and I could never understand how they worked.

Once out of school and working in technology, I bought a cat. When the lady asked why I wanted it, I told her I needed a bit of chaos around the house. The cat provided that chaos in a big way. Then I got married.[1]

For our first real date, I invited Sandy to go ice skating. We got to the rink, rented some skates, and then she told me she had never been ice skating. I told her I hadn't been either and offered a suggestion.

"Why don't we go out there and I'll hold you up, you hold me up, and we'll see how that works."

So we go out there on the ice. I'm holding onto her real tight so she doesn't fall, and she's holding onto me the same way. We went round and round. We probably looked strange to others at the rink; but it was so exciting to explore this intimacy that the path to the altar from that was quite short. I had been willing (as well as Sandy) to take that risk, to step out beyond my comfort zone, and to experience the adventure of doing something I had never experienced before no matter where it led. We went through life holding on to each other like that.

After we married we did a Marriage Encounter, learning a lot about how to communicate and express our love for one another. For example, I could come home from work and find her tinkering in the kitchen. I might ask what was for supper. She might say "pig's button hominy." That was a coded message she wanted to go out for dinner. I might ask her where she wanted to go, and she'd say it didn't really matter. At one level she really didn't care, she just wanted some intimate time with me. At another level she did care. I had to learn to discern what type of restaurant was in her vision for dinner. And she's not going to tell me. We had our own language. We had our own places where we would go when we wished to strengthen our intimacy. For the first time in my life I learned what unconditional and perfect love was.

I could misplace something and she could find it. She would watch me get all torqued out searching for it, then gently tell me to sit down, relax, have patience, and she would find it. And she would—and I'm the one who lost it!

This still goes on even after she has left to be with Jesus. One day after losing her I was taking a lady to hear a Bill Moyers' lecture on healing. On the day of the lecture, I couldn't find the tickets. I searched every stack of stuff in the house for hours and could not find those tickets. The lecture was sold out, but my tickets were lost. Finally, about mid-afternoon, I sat down (as Sandy would have me do) and prayed. First, I told God I needed those tickets and I couldn't find them. If he checked with Sandy, Sandy could tell him my language might get a little more colorful as I got more frustrated (no cursing, you understand, just borderline stuff). I told God to check with Sandy up there, as Sandy would know where the tickets were. I had a witness.

> *"Therefore we also, since we are surrounded by so great a cloud of witnesses, let us lay aside every weight, and the sin which so easily ensnares us, and let us run with endurance the race that is set before us,…"*
>
> —Heb 12:1–2 NKJV

In less than a minute after praying, I found the tickets in the first place I looked, the output tray of my copying machine under a stack of stuff. Now I hadn't copied the tickets, and even if someone else had they wouldn't be in the *output* tray of the machine *under* a stack of stuff.

The moral of the basic narrative here is that the intimacy with Sandy was still there. Through love, it acts even beyond the veil of death.

Now let's look at the real story of the parable. The ice rink is life itself. God asks us out on the ice with him and to accept all the risks involved. He's going to hold us up. He gives us a perfect, unconditional love. God only asks us to put *all* our weight on him. Accepting this invitation and stepping out on the ice is the first step in building intimacy with him. As we "dance" with him, we look strange to those about us. Yet we have found real healing, place, love, and purpose for the first time. We develop our own special language to talk with each other. We have our own special places we go to. The most important thing in life is this intimacy with God.

WE GAIN THE SIGNET RING

Read the story of Esther in the Bible. God asks her to step out on the ice, to go into the king's presence, and speak to save her nation. Get it? Here is a Jewish woman, a virgin, committed to God; and God is asking her to marry this Gentile heathen and then to go into the presence of this heathen king at the risk of her own life. To go before the king without being summoned by the king could mean death. Her reply to Mordecai who asks her to do it for God is simply "if I perish, I perish." Her action in stepping out saved the nation. She, in return, received the king's signet ring (or authority). She could now act in the name of the king.

As with Esther (and with Sandy and me), from our stepping out on God's invitation is born a rich intimacy. It is a rich, unconditional, and perfect love that God gives us. We can begin to understand his work-ing in our circumstances and claim his authority in the situation and healing. We are in the King's presence, he grants our desire, and then gives us the signet ring (authority) to act in his place. The signet ring was used by the king to sign letters. Her word became the king's word. In the same way, with this intimacy our word becomes the word of God and has his authority.

THE ROMANCE STORY

The story of my Sandy and the story of Esther are both romance sto-ries, sacred romances. In a far deeper sense, the entire Bible is also a romance novel. God will do anything to win our hearts. God also gives us the freedom of choice, just as he did with Adam, Moses, Esther, and the rest. Without that freedom to choose to love God, there can be no love on our part. We are designed for intimacy with him, and we are wounded without it. When Adam failed God, we inherited Adam's seed. That is, we failed God. So God came into our world and paid the price with the death of his Son so our freedom is restored. We, though, still have to choose. What love!

THE RISK

This intimacy with God begins with belief and ends with action. In the film *Indiana Jones and The Last Crusade* we see Indiana Jones (Harrison Ford) on a quest with his father (Sean Connery) for the Holy Grail, which is assumed to have healing powers. As they reach the end of the quest while pursued by the Nazis, Jones almost reaches the Grail but is separated from it by a large canyon. His father lies dying behind him, desperately needing a healing drink from the Grail. Jones sees no way to cross the massive canyon which seems infinitely deep. You then watch as Jones takes one step into the canyon and shifts all his weight to that foot with nothing but empty space under the foot. Jones risked everything. Suddenly a stone appears below his foot. Another step forward and another stone appears. Taking one step at a time, he reaches the Grail (and another test) before he takes the contents of the Grail back to his dying father and brings the healing he needs.

So often the healing we need is just as close as Jones was to that Holy Grail. To get to it, however, we have to take a step and a risk that seems beyond any reason. We have to put everything in the hands of God and trust him completely. The belief precedes the action. Without it, no healing will take place.

This belief can only be achieved through intimacy with God.

Dialogue

1. How did you feel when you watched that movie and saw Indiana Jones step out into the canyon?

2. In what way do you need to step out?

3. How can you make your prayer life better?

Notes

1. This is not an attempt to put down marriage or the issue of chaos. I had a wonderful marriage. The element of chaos in our life is becoming more interesting to scientists. It is from the chaos element that we can move in new directions outside of the rational and expected. A good leader generally initiates some level of chaos on those that follow to force them to think outside the boundaries. The followers who would not accept change under normal circumstances are forced to change. Sometimes I start the day with a prayer for God to do something wild (chaos to me) today. Then he does.

3

The Pursuit of the Heart

"To reveal one's heart and to lead from this in love is the highest form of leadership."

"All healing is first a healing of the heart."

All of us need healing. Jesus said he came not to the religious leaders but to those that needed healing and who could take the risk of releasing their heart to his authority in the healing. The religious leaders needed healing, but they could not release their heart to His authority. Healing is basically a heart issue. Both God and the Enemy struggle for our hearts. The healing of the heart must precede physical or emotional healing.

LETTING GO OF THE PERSONAGE

Many years ago one of the most outstanding doctors of the century, Dr. Paul Tournier, lived and ministered from his home in Switzerland. He was so successful that doctors all over the world often sent patients to him that they could not heal, only to see the patient successfully healed after they spent time with Dr. Tournier. Sometimes the doctors would ask Dr. Tournier how he did it, attempting to learn from his success.

The answer was quite simple, and Tournier published it in a book that was a watershed in my own life: *The Meaning of Persons*. In this book Tournier says we live in our roles and wear our masks for most of the day, sometimes even with our spouse. We are posers. To initiate the healing Dr. Tournier would invite the patient to his house. There, over coffee or tea and by the fireplace, the patients would drop their roles, games, and masks and share their true heart with Tournier. Tournier would often lead in the dialog, making his heart vulnerable to his patient. In so doing this encouraged his patient to open his or her own heart and be vulnerable. Tournier called the masked person the *personage*, the true heart and soul that must be touched for healing was the *person*. No healing can take place until this *person* is unmasked and revealed. We are all posers to some extent. All healing is first a healing of the heart.

In the movie *Groundhog Day*, we see Phil (Bill Murray) as the poser, earnestly seeking the heart of Rita. He's having the worst day of his life—over and over. Every morning he wakes up it is Groundhog Day, repeating all over again. He's stuck in a rut and can't get out. The only way he can get out of his small story and win the hand of Rita is to let go of the personage and his posing. Isn't that like us?

Our culture seems to divide the person into a physical, mental, and spiritual being and sends the person who needs help to a specialist in one of these areas. In reality, Dr. Tournier said, we are only *one* person, created in the image of God, and for true healing we have to see ourselves as *person*, a unique being that stands before God and is constantly in need of a healing process until we eventually meet the One who created us.

For most of us, there is always a part of us we reject. We wish we were as smart as so-and-so. We wish we had the handsome looks of some movie star. A pastor wants to preach like another one he knows. Maybe we wish we weren't crippled, blind, or perhaps living in a wheelchair. We fail to see that God created us just like we are from a vision he had for a unique purpose not "just before we were born," but from the beginning of time.

I've noticed that the better doctors always ask me questions about my job, my church life, and even the women I date. All of this is related to my physical well-being. One doctor told me over 85% of his patients come to him with stress-related problems. To begin their healing, he needs to know the cause of this stress. Doctors now say that if you are depressed, you are more likely to have a heart attack. The converse is also true. If the doctor says you are in danger of a heart attack, you will be depressed. You set yourself up for a heart attack from your emotional paradigm.

Scientists are making remarkable conclusions as they study the human genes. Genes are not, they have discovered, some immutable things handed down from our parents like Moses' stone tablets, but are active participants in our lives, designed to take their cues from everything that happens to us from the moment of conception. Nothing is hard-wired. Learning and education expands our capacity to choose our own path.[1]

I experienced what Tournier said years later as I sat in a workshop of men led by John Eldredge. Hurting and wounded from the loss of my wife and my own near fatal disease, John spoke incredible words to my heart. After the session, we broke into small groups. Within very few minutes, every man in that group was sharing at his deepest level of pain. Men don't do that. They will talk football, basketball, or golf, but for a man to make himself vulnerable looks wimpy. I was astonished. How did Eldredge do this?

The answer was simple, but the full depth of what John did was something I had yet to learn. John had lost his best friend and mentor only a few months before our conference. His friend had helped him author the book he was teaching us. John was very vulnerable to us about this and the struggle for the healing of his own heart from this. Yet this man I saw teaching us was strong, a leader, and was leading me to a place I hadn't been before!

When the men returned from this retreat, the wives saw an extraordinary change in their husbands. They wanted to know who this guy was and how he had done this. They begged the sponsoring church to bring Eldredge back so *they* could hear him. The next year the church did this, and again we all joined the journey and embraced the adventure. The third year Eldredge returned again, and this time the church needed to distribute tickets for those who wished to attend. The tickets were free, but were used as a method of crowd control. People took the tickets and distributed them to friends who were hurting. The church ran out of tickets but still let those who came attend the conference. Today Eldredge has thousands of men waiting to attend his conferences. Each of his books sells about a half-a-million copies or more.[2] Men no longer want to be posers. The church needs them as stallions, willing to face their wound and take the risk of being healed and healing others.

THE WOUNDED HEALER

The point here is that vulnerability, in a man, is not a sign of weakness. For a man or woman, to reveal one's heart and to lead from this in love is the highest form of leadership. The leader becomes invisible, and the follower is compelled to follow. We can only lead where we have been before, so the hurts, pains, and sufferings of this life are God's way of building intimacy with us and preparing us for leadership from *his* agenda.

I like the story Wayne McCroskey in my church told me about David and Goliath (after ministering to his wife through multiple surgeries).

> *"Then he took his staff in his hand; and he chose for himself five smooth stones from the brook, and put them in a shepherd's bag, in a pouch which he had, and his sling was in his hand. And he drew near to the Philistine."*
>
> —1 Sam 17:40–41 NKJV

"Do you know why David chose round stones instead of the other rough stones for his battle with Goliath?" he asked.

"No, I'd never thought about that," I confessed.

"A rough stone would not go straight to its mark. The sharp edges of a rough stone would catch the air and the flight of the stone would not be true. Only the smooth stones would go straight and strike Goliath at the one point he was vulnerable."

The stones David chose were smooth because they had weathered the years of being tossed about in the stream. Just so, as we are tossed about in life, God is preparing us for spiritual warfare and leadership. As a result, our prayers, discernments, and giftings become true and our intimacy with God deeper. We then become the weapon that God needs for the battle to establish his Kingdom. We should rejoice that we have been chosen for this. As my friend Sondra Hampe says, "Don't waste your trials."

There is another insight here in this story of David. Although the scripture doesn't explicitly say this, in all probability David knelt by the brook to select those stones. David, in kneeling by the brook for the stones, made himself vulnerable to the enemy. Yet this was an authentic action for him. Before kneeling, he had tried on Saul's armor. When he put on Saul's armor and staggered around in it young David made himself *really* vulnerable. It may have seemed right to those about him; but it was unauthentic, a personage that did not work for David. With the armor, David would have been a poser. David knew what did work for him, as he had used the slingshot to protect his sheep. He took off the armor, took only the smooth stones and his slingshot, and went into battle as an authentic man.

(Incidentally, Wayne also told me why David chose five stones when the first was all he needed to kill Goliath—Goliath has four brothers. Just kidding.)

We lead and heal from our own woundedness and authenticity. We are all wounded healers. Healing begins as we discover and reveal our heart to the one true healer.

Dialog

1. Watch the movie *Groundhog Day*. What changed with Phil so that he could move forward with his life? How does that apply to you?

2. Where are you a poser?

3. What does the phrase "God is pursuing your heart" mean to you?

Notes

1. Ridley, Matt. "What Makes You Who You Are". *TIME*, June 2, 2003, pp. 55—63.

2. Eldredge, John. *Wild at Heart: Discovering the Secret of a Man's Soul*. (Thomas Nelson Publishers: Nashville) 2001.

4

Daring to Pursue the Healing

"Do you want to be made well?"

—John 5:6b NKJV

*"Can't live with it, can't live without it. Sometimes it seems that humanity has **chosen** pain. In fact, we choose it every day."*

—Chris Seay and Greg Garrett, *The Gospel Reloaded*

Your ears are open but you don't hear a thing.
Your eyes are awake but you don't see a thing.
The people are blockheads!
They stick their fingers in their ears so they won't have to listen;
They screw their eyes shut so they won't have to look,
so they won't have to deal with me face-to-face
and let me heal them.

—Matt. 13:14b–15 *The Message*, Jesus quoting Isaiah 6:9–10, emphasis added

Do you want to be healed? Do you desire this with a passion? How much do you want to be healed?

The question reminds me of the story of someone who came to the pastor's wife of the church I was in during the sixties and asked how much it cost to be a member of that church. This lady had experienced so much healing that she wanted to give something back. The pastor's wife replied that it really didn't cost anything. The lady insisted. She wanted to pay something. Finally, the pastor's wife blurted out.

"Look, it really doesn't cost anything. But if you stay around long enough, you will find it costs you everything you've got."

This healing may cost you everything you've got.

Later, I was leaving this church and area for another job. I sat with the pastor and asked how I would be able to bring some of the healing journey I was experiencing in this church to my new church in the new location.

"Whatever God is asking you to do," he said. "embrace it with a passion. Pull a small group around you that believes in the vision with you. Then live into your passion as if your life depended on it. It may; but nothing else has any meaning. You may be rejected by the new church you are in, as change is often dangerous. The pastor and elders may not follow you. Stay with it, however. If you can't find a church for this, make it yourself."

AN EARLY HEALING PURSUIT

I did exactly that, following his advice to the letter. A small group of us in a larger church formed a small group and began to explore what "being a church" was all about. I remember a lady in our group who was particularly frustrated, saying the church wasn't relevant any more. I grabbed a polystyrene cup, wrote "church" on it, and then tore it to shreds. I then handed the pieces to her, asking her to put it back together. Our little group sat in silence as this very creative and artistic lady put it back together in a new form. Healing had begun for each person in the group. We were running on our passions.

From this bonding, we soon formed a small media group, taking skits and folk music to our church, other churches, and even a military base. I remember at a Chicago church we led a workshop experience. The older people in the church were worried because their kids were leaving the church. The first night of the workshop I grabbed a wastebasket, labeled it "church," and then stuck my foot in it and staggered onto the stage dragging this thing with me. When someone asked what was wrong, I explained that the church was holding me back and continued limping.

We loved it. We were all running on the edge of creativity and passions with a radical humor that cut across any current assumptions. Our budget was near zero. To get material, we got involved in outreach—people, the environment, politics, and everything else. The pastor supported us. The educational director of the church was in our group. I eventually married a girl who was a part of the group.

Healing can cost us everything we've got. As with this comment from the pastor's wife, the reference isn't just financial. If we don't rest in the journey, however, nothing else has any meaning. It is a risk we have to take to be healed, regardless of the cost.

THE MAN BY THE POOL

In John 5 we see a wonderful story of a man with an infirmity of thirty-eight years lying by the Pool of Bethesda.[1] The legend was that periodically the waters were disturbed by an angel. When this happened, the first person into the water would be cured. With a large group of people hovering around the pool and waiting for the next disturbance, Jesus chooses to come up to this one man.

> *"When Jesus saw him lying there, and knew that he already had been in that condition a long time, He said to him, 'Do you want to be made well?'"*

—John 5:6 NKJV

What a stupid question! It wasn't. If the man is healed, he will need to get a job, become a productive member of society. He could no longer depend on government dole. He would no longer be able to depend on others. He'd have to take charge of his life. I know of people like this. They don't want to get well, even with the pain they are living in.

The man replies in terms of the rational mindset of the people there, telling Jesus he has no one to help him to the pool, and when he gets there someone is always there before him. The man is in a small story with his rational and cultural boundaries. Isn't that like us? Jesus tells him to take up his bed and walk; that is, Jesus is telling the man to step outside of his small story and rational boundaries. Jesus heals him with nothing more than the spoken word. Notice something very important here, however: the man was obedient. He did exactly what Jesus told him to do. That's really the first step.

THE BIG QUESTION

If you study the Gospels, you will see that the question Jesus asked here is the basic question that Jesus often asked and that he asks it over and over again:

"What do you want me to do?"

You will find Jesus asking the same question to others in Luke 18:41, Matt. 20:21, Matt. 20:32, and Mark 10:36. In other healings Jesus often asks the same question, but indirectly, such as the story of the woman at the well. In other cases, people can't answer because they are mute or because they are controlled by demonic spirits. Read the scripture verses above and see if you can identify the common aspect of each story. In each case, Jesus was trying to reach out and meet the desires of the *heart*. Sometimes the desire was wrong, but the heart of Jesus was not. Jesus really wants to meet the deepest desires of our heart. We confuse our needs and our desires.

It is like the story my pastor told of the man who gave his wife a special gift for her birthday.

"Oh, it's just what I needed," she said, "to exchange for something I want."

Isn't that like us?

If Jesus has rich, deep spiritual discernment as to the needs of the people he met, why does he ask the question of what do we want when he knows? The answer is simple: We have to acknowledge our need to Jesus. *He has to hear from us that we desire the healing and can't do it on our own.* The Pharisees could not ask for this.

Another way to ask this question is what is your passion? What makes you come alive? What would you do if you were not limited by time, physical challenges, or financial resources? What adventure would you like to go on? What battle would you like to fight?

There are clues to this all about you. What movies have you seen that moved you? Perhaps you shared something about the movie with your friends. What was it you shared? Is that a clue? What books have you read that moved you? Why? What recent event (in your life or in the world) captivated your hidden heart and gave you some healing?

Jesus wants to meet the deepest desires of our heart. Of all the creatures God created, it is only Man that carries this deep longing in his heart for an adventure so deep and pure that he cannot express it, even to those who are closest to him. Somehow, however, in his prayers to the One who created him he begins to understand at least a little that he is heard and his desires will be met. As the Psalmist says:

> *"Delight yourself also in the LORD,*
> *And He shall give you the desires of your heart."*
>
> —Ps. 37:4 NKJV

or, in the words of Jesus:

> *"Until now you have asked nothing in My name. Ask, and you will receive, that your joy may be full."*
>
> —John 16:24 NKJV

Note: There is a caveat here. Jesus says we must ask *in his name.* Then again Jesus said:

"Have faith in God. For assuredly, I say to you, whoever says to this mountain, 'Be removed and be cast into the sea,' and does not doubt in his heart, but believes that those things he says will come to pass, he will have whatever he says. Therefore I say to you, whatever things you ask when you pray, believe that you receive them, and you will have them."

—Mark 11:22–24 NKJV

Or, as Andrew Murray said:

"God's giving is inseparably connected with our asking."

THE GREAT VISION STATEMENT

Ever thought about what Jesus' vision statement was? Nope, it's not the Great Commission. That's a mission statement telling who, what, when, where, and why. The vision statement of Jesus is back in Matt. 11:4–5. John was in prison and depressed. He sends his disciples to Jesus to ask if he really is the Messiah or should they look for another. Not a bad question, considering where John was and the reality that he would soon be beheaded. The reply of Jesus was his vision statement.

"Jesus answered and said to them, 'Go and tell John the things which you hear and see: The blind see and the lame walk; the lepers are cleansed and the deaf hear; the dead are raised up and the poor have the gospel preached to them.'"

—Matt 11: 4–5 NKJV

This story is also repeated in Luke 7:22.

At another time Jesus stood in the synagogue and read this much of the same statement from Isaiah 61, proclaiming that this prophecy was now fulfilled in their eyes.

> *"'The Spirit of the LORD is upon Me, Because He has a*
> *Me To preach the gospel to the poor; He has sent Me to h*
> *brokenhearted, To proclaim liberty to the captives And recovery of*
> *sight to the blind, To set at liberty those who are oppressed; To pro-*
> *claim the acceptable year of the LORD.'*
>
> *Then He closed the book, and gave it back to the attendant and*
> *sat down. And the eyes of all who were in the synagogue were fixed*
> *on Him. And He began to say to them, 'Today this Scripture is*
> *fulfilled in your hearing.'"*

—Luke 4:18–22 NKJV

Jesus is announcing that he has come to bring us freedom and release us from the bondage that has held us captive from the time of Adam and Eve.

But what Jesus said later about our role in this vision statement is even more startling:

> *"Most assuredly, I say to you, he who believes in Me, the works*
> *that I do he will do also; and greater works than these he will do,*
> *because I go to My Father. And whatever you ask in My name,*
> *that I will do, that the Father may be glorified in the Son. If you*
> *ask anything in My name, I will do it."*

—John 14:12–14 NKJV

This implies that not only does Jesus want us healed, but he wants to use us to heal others *in his name*. What an awesome thought! We have the responsibility of letting God use us to bring his Kingdom on earth! In addition, Jesus gives in this verse the reason why the healing will take place—to glorify the Father.

DO YOU WANT HEALING?

Some years ago I attended a prayer retreat at a remote area in Canada. After the retreat, I was sharing my testimony with a lady. I was sharing with her that in 1989 I was suddenly paralyzed from the shoulders down over a period of about 24 hours. I was in Switzerland at the time, and after a few weeks was flown back to the states, still paralyzed. The doctors told me here I would never walk again. Eventually I could walk again, without the wheelchairs or any other aid. I had only a small limp. I held a strong vision of wellness, of walking again, and acted into that vision.

The lady was amazed.

"That's a miracle," she said.

"Yes," I said. "God did it. Praise God!"

"You want the rest of it?" the girl said.

"What?"

"Do you want the rest of the healing?"

"Yes."

"Have you asked God?"

"No. I've prayed for others, but not for myself."

"Then how do you expect to be healed?"

This is where most of us are. It wouldn't be rational for me to be healed. The nerves were destroyed. I had bought into the myth of rationalization. Nerves don't grow, yet I had already experienced a tremendous level of healing. The nerves did grow! I was walking, even though the doctor said I would never walk again. God had already violated a few laws with the healing, and I had refused to believe he could do the rest if he wanted to do it.

In the hospital and paralyzed from the shoulders down, I had a strong passion to be healed. No one, not even the doctor, shared that passion with me. The doctor said I wouldn't walk again. The doctor wanted me to order two wheelchairs that I would need for the rest of my life. (I don't even use a cane now.) They would bring me catalogs of wheelchairs. Instead, I read the story of the healing of the lame man in Acts 3 each day. The psychologist had visited me and tried to help me get in touch with the reality of my situation. At the same time, I was witnessing to her trying to help her get in touch with the true reality of the situation.

Another time they put sensors on my ankles, picking up the pulse that went from the brain to the foot when I tried to move it. The pulse on the screen went off the screen, but the foot didn't move.

"How did you do that?" the doctor asked.

"Want to see it again?" I replied, shooting another pulse off the screen.

"Wow." she said. "If you could get out of here on will power, you'd be out of here today."

I turned to Sandy.

"See?" I said. "She says there's a way to get out of here today."

I had to live into that passion of *desiring* to be healed daily, and nothing else had any meaning to me. I would read the story of the lame man of Acts 3 daily. How did Peter do that? I did aggressive therapy twice a day. *My heart was my own; no one could heal it but Jesus.* The issue was strictly an affair of the heart. Healing is always an affair of the heart. There is a war going on. The war is for our hearts.

John Eldredge, in his book *Wild at Heart*, tells of a picture drawn by his nine-year old son.[2] The picture shows an angel in full armor, holding a two-handed sword, with his gaze steady and fierce. The kid had scrawled underneath the warrior in his childlike handwriting: "Every man is a warrior inside. But the choice to fight is his own." It is as if John is saying we must be a child to understand.

For me, after almost two months in the hospital paralyzed from the shoulder down they did a test to see if the nerves were being repaired. After the tests the top neurologist in the hospital came and stood by my bed with this puzzled look on his face. I asked him what the tests had shown.

"We don't understand," he said. "We've previously done the treatment you got in Switzerland here in the United States, but it doesn't work. Even in this case, the virus is still there. Yet your therapy results are showing continued healing even with the virus there. We don't understand, so we'll just keep on doing the therapy and what we have been doing."

I WANT TO SEE!

Some time ago a quiet, unassuming man came through Portland with a healing gift and stayed with some members in a church pastored by Rick, a friend of mine. Together this man and Rick went to the hospital and prayed for a kid who was scheduled for surgery the next day. Coming back from the hospital, they stopped at a coffee house.

"I want to pray for your eyes," the healer said.

Rick had always been color blind. His wife had to put his clothes out each day, as he could not color-coordinate them and was often embarrassed as a younger boy because he could not match things.

The healer prayed for him. The prayer was brief and lacked any particular drama. Rick said it was not accompanied by any faith or expectation on his part. Rick, however, was instantly healed of his color blindness. When Rick opened his eyes, a neon sign in front of him seemed to be exploding. Rick remains healed of his color blindness, and enjoys the sunsets and other sights he is seeing for the first time. Now imagine what that did in the church Rick pastors!

Like Rick, the blind Bartimaeus, and the servants of Elisha that could not see the army of the Lord—we all want to see!

> *"What do you want me to do for you?' Jesus asked him.*
> *The blind man said, 'Rabbi, I want to see.'"*
>
> —Mark 10:51 NIV

"And Elisha prayed, and said, 'LORD, I pray, open his eyes that he may see.' Then the LORD opened the eyes of the young man, and he saw. And behold, the mountain was full of horses and chariots of fire all around Elisha."

—2 Kings 6:16–18 NKJV

Where are you in these stories? Do you have self-imposed boundaries or bindings on the healing you desire? Can you identify these? How can you eliminate them? I will give you a clue: the most common bindings are unforgiveness and anger.

THE VISION OF WELLNESS

In the story of the lame man by the temple gate in Acts 3, there is apparently no vision on the part of the man. The man did not expect to be healed. He was forty years old, he had never walked, and after the healing he was running about, shouting and praising God. This is quite remarkable when you consider walking and running are learned experiences and the muscles would have never developed after his forty years of living without using them. There was no denial of the healing, as even the religious leaders who were upset about it could not deny it. How could this happen?

First, the healing is claimed by Peter in the name of Jesus, not from Peter's own authority. God had a vision for healing. The Holy Spirit used Peter to carry God's vision to the lame man. The man himself had no vision for healing. Peter had the faith to take the risk. Second, the purpose of the healing was to build up the Church and to glorify God. It had nothing to do with whether the man had a vision or not.

We know now from our scientific research that if we hold a vision of wellness it affects the immune system. The immune system is stronger. It will even affect the doctor caring for us. If he sees us wanting to be well, it encourages him or her and they will commit more of their resources to helping us. Almost any religious flavor can give us vision and appear to bring the healing, as it psychologically affects our belief that we will get well. The true healing, however, that reaches beyond the range of rationalization, is in the name of Jesus. Jesus made it plain that no man came to the Father (God) except through him.

The healing process, then, actually starts in the mind with the vision of wellness. The behavior follows belief. I know several people without jobs right now as I write this. Many of these are quite skilled, but their attempt over and over again to try to find a job has produced a mindset in which they believe they will lose the job opportunity even as they prepare their resume again and perhaps go for another interview. And they do fail. To win the job, they must believe this is a God-given job opportunity and go to the interview not just believing this (holding the vision), but also following through with their behavior doing things such as researching the company, finding out what the company really needs, and identifying how their unique skills fit this. In the final interview, the voice, posture, and appearance must witness to this confidence and personal vision.

For many, this is a difficult step. You are trying to bootstrap yourself, and with this bootstrapping process you never get higher than where your mentors and environment are. This means you have to release yourself to the Holy Spirit to give you the insights and power you need to turn the mindset around and map the successful strategy. Failure is not really a bad thing. Each time a resume fails you should learn something. What did you learn that will help you be more successful next time?

It is the same with our spiritual gifts. We may step out boldly, then fail. Learn from those who have traveled this way before. Risk again. I read of one man with an extraordinary gift of healing. He could pray for a person in a wheelchair and then watch them stand up and walk, never needing that chair again. Only thing was, it only worked for about one out of ten people for whom he prayed. For the others, he had to apologize publicly and then go on his way. Embarrassing? Sure, but he's way ahead of a lot of people I know.

One of my personal joys is to try to spend time with very creative people with rich spiritual insights as they cross my life. The dialog with them that I choose is not about their theology, but rather their journey to creativity, *which almost always includes much pain and suffering.*

THE STORY OF THE SAMARITAN WOMAN

Remember the story in the Bible of the Samaritan woman (see John 4)? This is an incredible example of how to communicate and draw a person to a salvation experience. Jesus targets the deepest needs of the woman and in very few sentences strikes at her needs, pulling her in, and initiating the healing. What did Jesus tell the woman she had to do to be released from her guilt?

Most of the women of that time came to the well in the evening to get their water. This woman came at noon. She was experiencing guilt about her life, and rejected by other women in the village. She was also rejected by men, as she had already been married five times. She came alone when she hoped no one else would be there. Jesus discerned her rejection. Jesus was a Jew, and Jews considered the Samaritans as half-breed heathens who had forsaken their faith in marrying spouses who were not Jews.

Jesus didn't give her a theology lesson or do what we commonly call evangelism by thrusting something on her and asking her to make a decision. Jesus did something remarkably simple. Jesus asked her for a drink. For Jesus, getting a drink would have been no problem. Jesus, however, had another reason for asking her for the drink.

This guilt-ridden woman without any sense of self-value seemed very surprised that a Jewish man would ask such a question of her. Here was a Jewish man (Jesus) who accepted her. Jesus was accepting her, giving her a personal sense of value.

She begins by trying to engage Jesus in what looks like a theological discussion.

"Where do we worship, here or at Jerusalem?"

This was not a theological question. She was really asking a deeply spiritual question. She had a deep yearning for something long lost. In asking where to worship, Jesus could hear her true passion. Jesus cut through this to the *heart of her desires*. There was a hunger there, a deep desire, and Jesus could discern this.

What Jesus did was appeal to her thirst, this deep desire of her soul. There was a passion for healing here, and Jesus spoke into her heart and initiated the healing. She didn't have to "do" anything except release her heart to the One who could heal her.

IS HEALING ALWAYS EXPERIENCED?

If God is good (and he is), why do those that love him suffer? This is a theological debate that goes back even before the life of Jesus. All of the disciples except one (John), if legends are correct, died as martyrs to their faith. Even as I write this, over 3000 are presumed dead in terrorist strikes on the United States. Why would a good God permit that?

The Apostle Paul has a partial answer for this in Philippians:

> *"Be anxious for nothing, but in everything by prayer and supplication, with thanksgiving, let your requests be made known to God; and the peace of God, which surpasses all understanding, will guard your hearts and minds through Christ Jesus."*
>
> —Phil. 4:6–7 NKJV

The physical healing may not be there, but another and deeper type of healing does take place. An extraordinary peace is there. That's the promise!

And then there is the promise in James:

> *"Is anyone among you suffering? Let him pray. Is anyone cheerful? Let him sing psalms. Is anyone among you sick? Let him call for the elders of the church, and let them pray over him, anointing him with oil in the name of the Lord. And the prayer of faith will*

save the sick, and the Lord will raise him up. And if he has com-
mitted sins, he will be forgiven. Confess your trespasses to one
another, and pray for one another, that you may be healed. The
effective, fervent prayer of a righteous man avails much."

—James 5:13–16 NKJV

In this verse, "will raise him up" is translated from the Greek word *egeiro*, which translates as to awaken, as from sleep or disease. The phrase "will save" is from the Greek word *sozo*, which means to heal, preserve, or make well. A few weeks ago a pastor in our church called me with the news someone in our church had been sick over a month with some virus the doctors could not even name. The best they could do was to give him steroids, which is really a very crude approach. We got a group of elders and went over. We read this verse together and made sure he believed it and knew of no sin he needed to confess. Then we prayed and anointed him with oil, claiming the authority and power (*rhema*) of the words in this verse. Six days later he was at a men's breakfast and almost completely healed, and the next day in our service we praised God for it.

God's purpose is not to make us happy, but to draw us to him and for us to experience intimacy with him. When the income is good and we are healthy, we often become more self-reliant and feel we have less need of God. The Apostle Paul had a gift of healing that was so intense that people could be healed walking in his shadow, yet Paul experienced deep pain for at least three people that he could not heal. Trophimus was left sick at Miletus by Paul (2 Tim. 4:20). Epaphroditus was ill and almost died (Phil. 2:26–27), and Timothy had a persistent stomach disorder in which Paul could only recommend a little wine. Paul himself suffered had a "thorn in the flesh" that defied healing in this life. Yet on Malta, he prayed and everyone who was sick was healed (Acts 28:9).

God's purpose in the suffering that we experience is to draw us closer to him. We should praise God for our trials, as they help us to know him better. The healing is always experienced, but sometimes not in the way or time frame we desire. Needs, desires, and God's agenda are often different things. There is, however, a certain fallacy in believing that God makes us sick in order that we can love him better. What father or mother would wish that on their child? We are made in God's image (Gen. 1:26), God is constantly remaking us in this image (2 Cor. 3:18), and one day in the future we will be perfect in his image (Phil. 3:20–21). Just as salvation is a present imperfect process (1 Peter 1:6–9), so is the healing. We will come back to this question later, looking at it from another perspective.

I have an advertisement from a magazine that I love. It shows a dark sky with a terrible tornado heading toward the viewer. Beside the tornado is a simple caption: "Looks like great surfing weather coming our way." That's a good summary of some spiritual experiences I've had.

Someone once asked Darby Conley, who draws the *Get Fuzzy* cartoon, what was his favorite. (This is the cartoon with the guy and his loser dog and egomaniac cat.) Darby said his favorite was the one with Sachel, the dog, happily eating a sandwich in the kitchen. Sachel suddenly notices something on the counter. When he leans over to look at it, he sees a bottle cap. On the cap he reads the words "You are not a winner" printed inside. Not understanding what that means, he becomes deeply depressed.

Isn't that like us? The world around us constantly tells us we are not a winner. We become depressed, sick, and fail to claim the wellness that God has for us.

In the story of Job in the Bible we see another story about healing. Job had the same question that we often have. Why doesn't God heal? There is a clue at the end of Job 3 where Job says:

"That which I feared the most has come upon me."

Job was still under the authority of God. Satan had to ask God for permission to test Job. God uses the trial to bring Job face-to-face with the one thing that Job feared the most. Perfect love casts out fear, and in this experience God is using his love to move Job beyond that fear.

Dialog

1. Read John 14:12–14. Do you believe that applies today? Why or why not?

2. What are some ways you can remove hindrances in your life that prevent your own healing and the healing of others you know?

3. Why do you think some people are not healed from a human viewpoint?

4. Is there anger or unforgiveness in your life that is blocking your healing? Have you asked God to remove this?

5. The verses in James 5 are a very bold statement. How do you interpret it? Are there conditions there for the healing?

Notes

1. The city of Bethesda, Maryland is named after this pool. The National Institutes of Health, a center of cutting edge medical research, is located there.

2. Eldredge, John. *Wild at Heart: Discovering the Secret of a Man's Soul.* (Thomas Nelson Publishers, Nashville). 2001. p. 140

5

Pursuing Deliverance Healing

"Having disarmed principalities and powers, He made a public spectacle of them, triumphing over them in it."

—Col. 2:15 NKJV

Most healing involves physical, spiritual, and emotional components. Jesus, in healing, was able to discern both the physical, spiritual, and emotional aspects of any healing and had authority and power in all areas.

JESUS AND THE DEMONIAC

To explore some of the issues of deliverance healing, let's take a look at the story of the healing of the Decapolis demoniac in the Gospels. This story is told in three Gospels. We will look at this story in this chapter and the next three chapters, so take a moment to read it in each Gospel:

Matt. 8:28–34

Mark 5:1–20

Luke 8:26–39

There are some differences in the story, but that does not affect the message here. You also need to go back and see the time line of what was happening. Jesus had been healing people on the west side of the Sea of Galilee. It was the Sabbath, and Jesus had already been at the

synagogue and healed a man with a demonic spirit. He had sent healing to a centurion's servant. Then he healed Peter's wife's mother. He
had met with opposition for his healing on the Sabbath.

Officially the Sabbath ended when two stars appeared in the sky.
We see a crowd coming to Jesus on the west side of the Sea of Galilee.
The Sabbath is over and it is now evening (Matthew says it was
evening), so already the stars were shining. Jesus continues to heal after
a long day. He is also teaching as he sits in a boat (Mark 4:1). Finally,
Jesus gives orders for the disciples to get in the boat with him and tells
them he plans to cross to the other side of the Sea of Galilee. Note that
Jesus has a specific agenda in mind. Jesus is moving *to* something, not
away.

With darkness already encroaching, Jesus decides to cross the Sea of
Galilee with his disciples to the Decapolis area. Jesus, tired from the
day, went to sleep in the boat. A storm arose on the sea. This was not
unusual for this Sea of Galilee. The surrounding mountains still act
today as a type of venturi effect where storms can come up suddenly on
the sea, putting small fishermen in their fishing boats in peril of their
lives. The same effect today is used in rockets, with a small constricted
area in the exit used to speed up the exit of the rocket's gases. This sea
is in a canyon, and the winds act much in the same way. The waves
would have been about twenty feet high, covering the boat (Matthew
8:24). The word used here in Greek indicates the boat was actually
hidden by the waves, with water coming into the boat. The word used
to describe the storm is *seismos,* from which we get the word for an
earthquake.

The disciples panicked as these twenty-foot waves swamped the
boat, afraid they would die. In the Jewish culture of that time, the
storm and the waves would have been considered demonic and attrib-
uted to Satan. I believe this truly was a demonic encounter. Jesus was
still asleep. The disciples woke him with their concern. They were
afraid they would perish. Jesus rebuked the storm telling it to be silent,
and immediately there was a great calm. (Jesus used the same words in

healing the demoniac in Mark 1:25.) Then Jesus chided the disciples about their lack of faith. Soon after that, they pulled to shore at the Decapolis area. The entire journey would be about five miles, so now it is late evening or perhaps even night.

THE DECAPOLIS AREA

The Decapolis area was an area around the shore of the Sea of Galilee.[1] The area consisted of ten cities ("Deca" means ten, "polis" means city.) These were primarily Greek cities, or Gentile. The Decapolis region was southeast of the Sea of Galilee and also swung slightly south and under the Sea of Galilee, with a small part to the west of the Jordan River. It was considered probably the darkest part (spiritually) of Palestine.

The ten Greek cities were Scythopolis, Dion, Pella, Gerasa, Philadelphia, Gadara, Raphana, Hippos, Kanatha, and Damascus. Scythopolis was most western, probably the largest, and the only one west of the Jordan. Philadelphia was the furtherest south and is the location of today's modern Amman. The cities were founded by Alexander the Great as he led the Greek penetration into Palestine and Syria. Although the cities were in Syria when founded, with Alexander's conquest they became Greek, but really independent. They had their own administration, their own commerce, coins, and defense system. They remained as fairly independent until the Maccabees conquered the area about the middle of the second century (B.C.) and put the cities under their Jewish rule. They were liberated from this Jewish rule about 63 B.C. by the Roman emperor Pompey.

At the time of Jesus the cities were now under Roman rule with Roman taxation and subject to the Roman military service. Unfortunately, Rome could give them little protection. So they banded together much as a federation to defend themselves from Arabian and Jewish encroachment. Culturally, they remained Greek with their

Greek gods, temples, baths, and amphitheaters. They were very beautiful cities.

Archeological diggings in the area have discovered the remains of pagan temples, forums, and other signs of the pagan Gentile culture. A few Jews lived here; but the Decapolis area was mostly Gentile. The fact that pigs are here indicates this had certainly very little Jewish influence and was very dark spiritually. The Luke account says this area was the opposite of Galilee. It is almost as if Luke is using a pun to refer to it being both geographically and spiritually opposite Galilee.

GOING ASHORE

Jesus and his disciples were coming ashore in the Decapolis area to what was certainly a cemetery. There are caves here, and these caves were used for burial purposes. The wild man in the story lived in the caves. It would be evening or probably night. If it was late twilight, the long shadows of the wild man moving across the cemetery would frighten anyone. If it was night and there was moonlight, the shadows of the man in the moonlight would have been moving about. If it was a dark night, they would have heard the man moving about and screaming, but would have seen nothing. There is no one else here except some swine herders on the remote hills. Jesus and his disciples were entering a very dark area—physically, emotionally, and spiritually. How would you feel entering a cemetery with a deranged man living there, screaming at you, and it is night? The disciples apparently say nothing.

THE DECAPOLIS IN YOUR LIFE

Where is this Decapolis in your life? If the question were asked of me, my immediate answer would be to think of the time I was with my wife in Seattle as she got a bone marrow transplant for her leukemia (she did not survive it). There is a cluster of hospitals there known to the locals as "pill hill." The death rate there is very high. It isn't that they do anything wrong, it is just that the hospitals are operating on the edge of medical technology. When we checked in, they told us her chance of surviving the transplant was 50%. If we decided to go home without it, her chance of surviving a year was 10%. We could choose. The doctors are only there three months—one month inpatient work, one month outpatient, and one month research. While I was there two patients died on one side of Sandy and one on the other. The nurses, however, remained. I asked a nurse how she was able to survive and work in such a difficult place.

"To see one kid alive after a year who would have certainly been dead without the transplant;" one nurse told me. "that keeps me going."

Patients often come in angry. Parents, spouses, and friends who visit are often angry as well. Many have no spiritual resources to cope with what they see. How could a loving God do this? The loss of a loved one or a child seems to have no meaning. A patient may go into a catatonic state for no apparent reason as doctors race around the clock with various tests to try to find out why. We have very little theology to understand this, and the academic excursions of the theologians have little meaning in this spiritual battlefield.

I remember one beautiful lady whom I saw coming back from the hospital to her apartment daily with a smile on her face, hope in her eyes. They were going to save her baby. The husband apparently was staying back home, working. It gave us hope to see her joy each day. Then one day she came back to the apartment and the smile was gone. The face was tear-streaked. She left the next day. I remember another hunky and extraverted football player there who had the transplant and stayed in an isolated room for weeks and no one could even touch him. His immune system would be gone during that time, and the doctors couldn't risk it. The isolation was psychologically destroying him, and the father was afraid he would go insane. At the same time you watch your loved one going through incredible pain because you want her to stay alive. She's doing it for you. Emotions race through you that you have never experienced before.

Nothing makes sense anymore. You are in your Decapolis. What are you going to do about it?

Actually, the real Decapolis in your life is much darker than this; but the Enemy doesn't want you to see it. (See Chapter 7).

THE ISSUE OF DELIVERANCE

Now let's take a look at the spiritual picture here of what is happening and how it relates to the issues of deliverance. Some Bibles give a terrible translation in Matt. 8:31 indicating that Jesus cast the "devils" out. Other versions imply the man was demon possessed, which again is not theologically correct. The man is owned and possessed by God, just as you are. God created everything and God owns everything. When Man sinned, the ownership didn't change. God still owns the man. God still owns you. You have authority to choose your destiny, however. This is much like an owner of an apartment renting you the apartment. The owner still owns the apartment, but you have the keys and the authority to use the apartment. You choose how you use the apartment. In the same way God still owns this man, but this man has released *authority* in his life to the evil spirits.

"For the world is Mine, and all its fullness."

—Ps 50:12 NKJV

The Greek word used here to describe this man's problem is *daimonizomai*, which means to be under the control of a spirit or spirit guide. A *daimon* was a spirit or spirit guide. In the Greek culture it could refer to any spirit, good or bad. Here in the New Testament Jesus uses *daimon* to refer to an evil spirit, or in this case multiple evil spirits. Jesus didn't cast the devil out. The Greek word for the devil is *diabolos*, which means the accuser. In John 13:2, it is the *diabolos*, or devil, that enters the heart of Judas as he leaves the supper to betray Jesus. The devil (of which there is one) sent the evil spirits (of which there were many) to influence (not possess) the man. Jesus casts out the evil spirits.

In Luke 9:1, Jesus gave the disciples the power (*dunamis*, to do) to cast out *daimonions*, or evil spirits (not devils, as some versions mistranslate). This was under the authority of Jesus, not the Holy Spirit. When Jesus was arrested, the disciples were not arrested, as they were not considered a threat at that time. After they received the power of the Holy Spirit in Acts, they did become a threat, an enigma to the culture around them. After all, smelly fishermen don't go around enabling a lame man of forty years to instantly walk (Acts 3).

This is not a story of a man bound by superstitions in a world long ago. It is real. In ministering to people today, the binding to evil spirits is often very real. In fact, I find people who don't know the Lord are often very afraid of even talking about the subject of evil spirits even as I sense where the demonic spirits have entered their life. Sometimes the binding is a very common type, such as a child afraid of the dark, a woman (who almost drowned once as a child) afraid of the water, or someone who fell from a horse afraid of horses. I remember the first time I fried chicken the grease caught on fire. I got burned, but once the incident was over I got some more chicken and fried it right the next time, and in doing so broke the binding. Sometimes, however, the binding can be deep and dark.

A woman with child may choose an abortion, only to change her mind and continue the pregnancy. The incident, however, has already sent a message to the unborn child, and a very real binding on both the mother and child will be there when the child is born. In another situation, a father may never really affirm or accept his daughter, binding her to a pattern that results in multiple marriages and divorces. A woman may finally escape an abusive marriage, only to find she has difficulty building intimacy with a man again because of the binding from the abuse in her previous marriage. A man can be destroyed by his father if the father sees him only as a wimpy boy (in terms of what the father expects of the son) instead of the stallion God has called the son to be.

Over and over again we see this bound man (or woman) in our culture today. Often in ministering to this person I have to trace back in time to find where the binding first came into the life, and it is not unusual to find it in a previous generation and passed on to that person carrying a curse from a previous generation.

In this type of ministry, the power of the Holy Spirit is always stronger than that of the evil spirits. The difficulty is often in discerning the spirits and their orchestration. Our job is to pray for discernment, then claim authority over them in the name of Jesus. We can rebuke the demonic spirits in the name of Jesus. For example, if a man comes to me and expresses guilt over an incident in his past, then asks for a strategy to release that guilt. The binding spirit here is the spirit of legality. He thinks that if he does something he will be free. As a Christian, however, this man is already free by the blood of Jesus.

I like the story Brennan Manning tells[2] of the woman who was having several apparitions in which Jesus appeared to her. An archbishop sought her out, as he was fascinated by the stories. The archbishop said he had some sins he had confessed, and he asked the woman that the next time she had the apparition to ask Jesus what these were.

Several days later the woman had another apparition and contacted the archbishop as he had requested.

"Did you do what I asked?" the priest asked.

"Yes," she replied. "I asked him to tell me the sins you had confessed in your last confession."

"What did he say?"

"Bishop," she said. "these are his exact words: 'I can't remember.'"

Dialog:

1. Where is the Decapolis in your own life?

2. Where is the Decapolis in your church? Your city?

3. We all have bindings on our life of one type or another. What bindings do you sense on your own life? How do you feel about these?

Notes

1. There is some confusion between the gospels on the number of wild men here and the actual location. Matthew places the incident in the country of the Gadarenes and says there were two men. Mark and Luke tell of one man in the country of the Gerasenes. The only Gerasa we know anything about was thirty-six miles inland and certainly isn't the location from the story we see here. Another town of Gadara was six miles inland, and was a possible location. Oriten, a great scholar of the third century, knew of a town Gergesa that was right on the shore of the sea and believed it to be the most likely location. The problem is probably in the copying of the early texts and the lack of knowledge by those who did.

2. Manning, Brennan. *The Ragamuffin Gospel.* (Multnomah Publishers: Sisters, OR). 2000. pp. 115–116

6

Breaking the Bindings

"Power never was and never will be the issue between God and Satan. Authority was the issue—the authority Satan had obtained through Adam. Jesus did not come to get back any power, nor to remove Satan's power. He came to regain the authority Adam lost to the serpent and break his headship over the earth…Authority is the issue. Power does the work, but authority controls the power… The power issue was won in heaven by God before man was created, and won on earth at the cross."

—Dutch Sheets[1]

As we look at the demoniac, we see something very astounding. Here was a man who was wild. He could not be bound with chains (Mark 5:3). Yet something was obviously binding this man, and it was stronger than chains. Whatever it was, he couldn't break loose of it. He could break the chains, but not whatever this was that was binding him.

What is binding you from experiencing the healing that God wants to give you? The Enemy wants you to think that you are powerless and brings accusations and discouragement. The truth is, God grants him some power, but that is delegated by God (see the story of Job). The Enemy's power is real, but (unlike God's) is limited.

Put yourself in the story as one of the disciples. You have just come across the Sea of Galilee and faced (at least in your mind) a demonic storm. You have just come ashore at a cemetery at night (when they thought the demons came out) and this naked wild man comes run-

ning at you and yelling. He is probably a Gentile, condemned to hell
already in the Jewish mind of the time. What would you do? How
would you see the man that is running at you? How did Jesus see him?

Remember the WWJD (What Would Jesus Do) bracelets? What
did the disciples do? It is apparent from the story that they said nothing, apparently caught up in the fear and awe, just like they had been a
few hours earlier on the Sea of Galilee in the storm. What did Jesus do?
He moved in with authority, just as he did a few hours earlier in the
storm. What would you do?

Dealing with Our Own Bindings

High on the highway to the cascade's Mt. Hood near me is a restaurant
I love to visit. Near the restaurant entrance you can see deep tracks in
some rocks. They were once a part of the Barlow Trail that carried the
pioneers over the mountain over a hundred years ago. The tracks are
petrified now, and one can only image the pain, cost, and loss of life as
those pioneers crossed the mountain. The actual passage the pioneers
used is now known as the "chute" and is nearby at Laurel Hill. The
pioneers would come up the trail with all their possessions rather than
risk the rapids of the Columbia River. They would put all of their possessions in their wagon, and tie a rope from the wagon to a tree on the
trail. After that they would lower the wagon down this west side of the
mountain by the rope until they had reached the canyon floor leading
to Oregon City. Sometimes the rope might break, possessions lost, or
perhaps they might experience death or injury from a runaway wagon.
Now the deep tracks stand mute with their story petrified in the rock.

How many of us are like that rock? Deep bindings from the past cut
across our lives, decade after decade. The wounds are deep, now petrified: The woman who fails at marriage again and again because she
never experienced any messages from her father and the men she married that she is esteemed, valued, and worthy of pursuit. The man who
cannot give himself to adventure, his personal battle, or intimacy with

a woman because he never heard from his father that he has strength for these. Stronger than chains, these ruts from the repeated behavior patterns keep us from experiencing the healing that God has for us. We live in our small stories, never willing to take the risk to move to the larger story beyond where we are.

Like this demoniac who stood before Jesus, you have a choice. What are you going to do about that choice? Are you a stallion or gelding?

DEALING WITH MY PERSONAL FEAR

I had just gotten a newsletter from Bob Waymire about six months after my wife's death and four years after my paralysis. There at the bottom Bob had scrawled:

"Let me know when you are ready."

I called him and laughed and said "What do you mean 'When I'm ready?'"

"Oh…Oh—travel again."

"I've been ready. Done some traveling. Where are we going?"

"London."

Silence. Bob continued, "You have a problem with that?"

Bob knew I had a problem with that. My last trip to London had been with Bob. That's where I had gotten the virus that ten days later left me paralyzed from the shoulders down and took me over a year to recover.

"Bob, I have a major problem. Nevertheless, I don't make the decisions. God does. I'll check with God and let you know."

The next day I'm sharing this with my pastor (Peter Batchelder at that time). I confessed my fears.

"That's no reason to give him a no," Peter said.

"Peter, you are no help."

Now I don't normally put out fleeces, but in this case God's going to have to give me some signs. For the first sign, the money has to be there. The next day there is a $50,000 royalty check for me in the mail.

Bummer. At the final count God had given me about 11 signs I was supposed to go.

They say that if you want to find God, go where God is working and let him take it from there. If I did that, England wouldn't even be on my long list. I had already made four trips there, and there was no sign of him except in the architecture, art, and music that spoke of past ages. I could sit in a church on Sunday morning in England with about six others and hear a powerful sermon that echoed in an empty room off of the stone walls.

Oops, one exception. Back in the sixties on a Sunday afternoon I got off a train in York and wandered over to an ancient cathedral in a pouring rain. There I found hundreds or maybe thousands in a standing-room-only service praising God.

So why did God want me to go now?

Then there was the shingles story about a month before the trip. I was diagnosed on a Thursday; I called Bob that Saturday to tell him the trip was off because I had the shingles. He was in a board meeting. They prayed. The shingles were suddenly gone that afternoon. On Monday the doctor confirmed it, giving me some antibiotics to get my immune system back up. The trip was back on.

As the date approached, my church decided they had better pray for me in a Sunday night service as the whole thing was getting weird. A friend of mine, who had some type of prophetic gift, came up to me quietly and told me, "Don't go alone."

"What does that mean?"

"I don't know. I'm just looking at Daniel 10, and the Lord is telling me for you not to go alone."

"Right."

The next day my ticket agent is calling me asking if I want to cut the London ticket. This day was the deadline.

"Yes," I said. "but cut two."

"What name goes on the other?"

"I don't know. Just put my name for now."

"That's double-booking. I can't do that."

The agent says she will put her name on the other ticket, but it has to be off by the end of the week, as she's leaving by then.

"OK, I should know the name by then."

The next morning I'm eating breakfast with Peter Batchelder, my pastor.

"I'm getting a weird word from the Lord," Peter says. "I think I am supposed to go with you and my wife confirms it. She's never confirmed anything that fast before."

"Peter, I've got the ticket cut."

Do you want to see a guy fall off his chair?

So there we were. Two guys going to London with Bob, and neither of us knows why we are going there. There's a *lot* more to this story, but you can see I'm trying to find light again when everything around seems to be in darkness and I'm heading into a territory where I lost the war the last time I was there.

The Lord set us down at a community known as the Ichthus Christian Fellowship. Here as a small community they were committed to changing the face of England and bringing the Kingdom there. This was the base for Graham Kendrick, the writer of that marvelous Christian song *Shine Jesus Shine*. This was also the base for Richard Foster, a primary leader in the March for Jesus movement. Foster was off with some pastors fasting and praying. C. Peter Wagner came in and out while I was there, checking on the thousands of points of light around the world for his research for the books he writes. Here at Ichthus they were feeding church data from all over England into their computers, and for the first time I could see maps on the computer that showed places in England where revival was already starting to break, and they could track church growth chronologically. In the shadow of St. Paul's Cathedral I had the opportunity to share with them about my years of work with spiritual mapping. In a small teahouse with Peter we shared with a man from Germany who had driven all night to dialog with me on starting his own mapping, asking me what was the most important thing about starting (a good prayer team). Somehow within the context of this community my fear vanished. I knew I was supposed to be there, a witness to the coming of the Kingdom. My fear was gone.

DEALING WITH FEAR

Now let's return to the story of the demoniac and the fear of the disciples as they entered the darkness there. As you read the story in each of the gospels, notice a common element. The disciples are silent. After the incident of the storm on the Sea of Galilee, it is as if they are paralyzed by fear as the rest of the story unfolds before them.

In Tolkien's *Lord of the Rings*, Frodo with the other hobbits leave the Shire and take the more dangerous route through the Old Forest instead of the open road, knowing that the Enemy was pursuing them. The forest was not only dark and foreboding; it was hostile and seemed bent on the destruction of the hobbits. Some of the hobbits are swallowed up by a tree. It is Tom Bombadil that rescues them and takes them to his house, where his wife, Goldberry, welcomes them.[2]

"Come, dear folk…Laugh and be merry…Let us shut out the night. Fear nothing!"

There in Tom's house they were surrounded by goodness with laughter, bread, meat, song, drink, and downy soft beds. Love and grace are poured out on them. Later, we find it is Tom who has the power and authority to rescue them from what would have been certain death in this same area.

> *"Then he [Nehemiah] said to them, 'Go your way, eat the fat, drink the sweet, and send portions to those for whom nothing is prepared; for this day is holy to our LORD. Do not sorrow, for the joy of the LORD is your strength.'"*
>
> —Nehemiah 8:10 NKJV

We live in a fallen world. Man was given dominion of the world by God at creation. The world was good as he made it (Gen. 1:31). When Man fell to Satan, the earth (subject to Man) fell to the Enemy as well. Jesus came to a fallen planet, died, and then rose in victory over this broken world.

Like Frodo and the hobbits, we tremble as the disciples did as we journey through the shadows of the Old Forest. If we don't, we don't know about the dangers of the journey and are asleep to the reality. Both God and the Enemy wrestle for our hearts.

The opposite of love is not hate, but fear.

> *"There is no fear in love; but perfect love casts out fear, because fear involves torment. But he who fears has not been made perfect in love."*
>
> —1 John 4:18 NKJV

The word "fear" is used 28 times in the gospels and the word "afraid" is used 31 times. The essential "Don't be afraid" is used over and over again in the Bible.

> *"Peace I leave with you, My peace I give to you; not as the world gives do I give to you. Let not your heart be troubled, neither let it be afraid."*
>
> —John 14: 27–28 NKJV

One young man brought to me for healing had just become a Christian and was now tormented by demonic spirits every night. Using my computer-based concordance, I first created a listing of all the verses that had to do with fear. Then I sat with the young man at his house and had him read from this list verse after verse about what Christ said about not being afraid. You could see his expression change as he read the verses until finally he asked.

"Is it OK if I dance?"

And he danced and danced and danced. We rejoiced and worshiped with him at the healing.

The bindings had been broken.

WHAT THE WINNING MOVIES TELL US

During 2002 three movies were released that drew phenomenal crowds, mostly kids:

- *Harry Potter and the Chamber of Secrets*

- *Spider-Man*

- *Star Wars Episode—Attack of the Clones*

What was the common thing in all three of these movies, and why did that make them so popular? In each of these movies, we saw a young man who never got the message from his father that he had strength for his adventure, battle, and pursuit that he was called to in life. Each of these young men went on with their lives, frustrated and bound by the lack of this message. Isn't that where so many young men are today?

With Harry Potter you see a young man who watched as his parents were murdered, then he was moved to a family that consistently sent messages to him that he had no value. This strange school of magic sees him as a hero, takes him in, and affirms his value and strength. No wonder these books sell in the millions and J.K. Rowling is the richest woman in England!

One Christian psychologist, when asked about these books, replied simply:

"I see Harry Potter in my office every day."

Do you see the pattern here?

There is a breaking up of the family in America, a lack of relevance of most churches for any authority and power in changing this, and very few core values. Both young men and young women are not getting the messages they need in order to see themselves with spiritual authority and power.

It wasn't that long ago that a few kids (very young) walked by a pornographic store near me and prayed for its destruction. Then they went on home, over an hour's drive away. That night the store burned down, and one man inside died in the fire. *These were kids who already had spiritual authority and power and were free of the bindings our culture so often imposes on them.* They had been raised by their parents without television, movies, schools teaching liberal humanism, and many other cultural influences. They didn't know what they did was not rational, and took spiritual authority and power to make it happen. They had no bindings.

WHAT THE BLACKBIRD TELLS US

Not too far from my house is an aviation museum that houses the famous Spruce Goose (a very large wooden plane built by Howard Hughes) and also one of the famous Blackbirds, or more technically an SR-71. Although this plane is dated now, at the time nothing—I mean nothing—could stop it. Flying at three times the speed of sound and at the threshold of space, it was almost impossible to detect. If you did detect it, you couldn't shoot it down because it was faster than anything you could shoot at it. The skin was made of titanium.

If you saw this plane fueled and ready for a flight, however, you would think it had major design problems. The skin doesn't fit right and it's leaking fuel all over the place. The pilot is sitting in what is really not much more than a massive fuel tank. The huge plane can only carry enough fuel to get into a flight, and must be refueled again as soon as it gets in the air. *But sitting on the ground is not what the plane is made for!* Once in flight, the titanium skin seals itself as it expands and the seals in the fuel line close. The titanium skin actually gets stronger with each flight as it heats to the high temperatures of about 600 degrees Fahrenheit at the cockpit when flying at Mach 3.

Isn't that the way we should be? Many people I meet are much like that SR-71 on the ground, frustrated and broken. But that's not what we are made for! We are designed to fly faster than the speed of sound, soaring to the skies, and getting spiritually stronger on each flight!

THE ESCAPE ARTIST

Graham Cooke helped birth a church in England in 1974 with a group of 35 students. They had their own Pentecost when the Holy Spirit hit them and are now 8000 congregations in 44 countries. One of these congregations in England is a street church that takes the gospel to the streets using jugglers, fire-eaters, illusionists, and an escape artist. Now this escape artist is really good. He gives a little spiel about how we are trapped by the Enemy (in our chaos, Decapolis,...), and then lets then lets the audience tie him up with a straitjacket, padlocks, chains, and more. The audience watches as he struggles to break loose, and he eventually gets free. Then a second guy comes up (rather overweight) and gives the same spiel. Again, they tie him up in the same way with a straightjacket, padlocks, and chains. Only he can't break loose, and just sits there describing all the bondages in his life. Then he starts crying. Cooke says this little group is leading more people to the Lord than any of their local congregations. Which guy are you?

Dialog

1. What bindings were on the disciples of Jesus? Where did those come from?

2. What bindings do you see that have been imposed on you?

3. Which bindings came from your parents?

4. Which bindings came from your culture?

5. How can you move beyond these?

6. In the section on the Winning Movies, the question was raised about the breaking up of the American family. How can you be a part of changing this and restoring the family?

Notes

1. Sheets, Dutch. *Intercessory Prayer: How God Can Use Your Prayers to Move Heaven and Earth.* (Regal: Ventura, CA). 1996. p. 153. This is a classic book about prayer. Be sure it's in your library.

2. Unfortunately, this story is omitted from the movie. You'll have to read the book to find it.

7

The Desire for Identity and Purpose

"It's in Christ that we find out who we are and what we are living for. Long before we first heard of Christ and got our hopes up, he had his eye on us, had designs on us for glorious living, part of the overall purpose he is working out in everything and everyone."

—Eph. 1:11–12 *The Message*

Some time ago I watched Larry King doing an interview with Ryan Corbin on King's television show. In reality, Larry King has done several interviews with Ryan and has followed him for over a year through Ryan's healing journey. About 18 months before the interview I watched, Ryan had a tragic fall that had left him paralyzed and barely able to speak. Ryan's grandfather, Pat Boone, was on the show as well with Ryan's mother and sister. The family was pouring out love on him, cheering him on, and Pat was even doing some singing with him. Slowly, the young man was beginning to get his life back. The young man's pastor was also there—Rick Warren, the pastor of Saddleback Church and the author of several books, including *The Purpose Driven Life*. Larry was dialoging with them on the question that haunts all of us at times: "Can you really see the purpose of God in this?"

Rick Warren's answer summed up our starting point: "A person can really go through anything as long as they can see the purpose in it." In reality, several people have already come to the Lord from Ryan's witness since his fall.

To experience healing, we must pray for God to reveal his purpose (*his* purpose, not ours). Embracing the purpose will lead us to another identity and name.

JESUS CHANGES THE IDENTITY OF THE DEMONIAC

When Jesus first approached the demoniac, we see that his first attempt to heal the man met with failure.

> *"For He said to him, 'Come out of the man, unclean spirit!'"*
>
> —Mark 5:8 NKJV

Notice that Jesus is calling the evil spirit by name. Nothing happened. Then Jesus did an interesting thing:

> *"Then He asked him, 'What is your name?'"*
>
> —Mark 5:9 NKJV

This man's name at that time represented his character, or identity. It represented the essence and heart of the person. Many times in the Bible we see a person's name changed as they accept God's call on their life. Abram became Abraham and Sarai became Sarah, Jacob (the trickster) became Israel ("He Struggles with God"). Simon became Peter (Rock), and Saul became Paul (a Gentile name, signifying his new calling). Jesus is preparing to change the identity of the demoniac. Now his identity is a wild man, the demoniac. Soon he will have a new identity that will be known through the years as "the man who was healed of demonic spirits." His identity will be changed. Jesus needs to know the name of the evil spirits in the man in order for Jesus to take authority over them.

In the story of the man by the Pool of Bethesda, Jesus also changed an identity, or name. When Jesus first met him, he was "the man with an infirmity by the Pool of Bethesda." After Jesus healed him, he became the "man who was healed of an infirmity by the Pool of Bethesda." That is all the difference in the world. In both stories, we see something happens (a healing) that we read about thousands of years later.

The new name is our mythic name. To quote David Whyte, it reveals what we are capable of. It brings healing. There is a transcendent quality to this mythic name that not only reveals who we really are, heals, but also empowers us to reach for that, even if it means our death. Look what happened in the Bible as Peter, Paul, and others took on their mythic names.

When you go to the doctor, what is the first question you have? Recently I went to the doctor because I was experiencing heartburn, often two or three times a day. He did some testing, and then told me I had Barrett's Esophagus, and without treatment I had a small probability of getting cancer there, although there was no cancer there at the present time. He put me on a specific medication that stopped the heartburn and prevented further damage. He also told me to return in two years for another checkup, sooner if I had problems.

In the naming of the disease, the doctor was able to take control (authority) over it. The vision of wellness that he gave me strengthened the immune system. Now I can experience wellness. There is no more heartburn.

It is the same in the spiritual dimension. Jesus, in naming the binding and wound, is able to take authority over it. Even if we don't know the name of it, we can ask the Holy Spirit to reveal the name to us. Then Jesus can take authority over it. We can pray in Jesus' name, strategically, for the healing.

THE IDENTITY ISSUE

For healing to take place:

• You must know the identity of Jesus

- You need to identify the name of what Jesus must take authority over. The Holy Spirit can reveal this.

Jesus at one point asks his disciples what they thought his identity was (Mark 8:27–30). To quote Graham Cooke, Jesus didn't have an identity crisis here; he just wanted to be sure the disciples didn't. The disciples (quoting the crowds) gave three distorted identities. When Jesus asks specifically who they think he is, Peter gives the correct identity. The question here, then, is who do *you* say that he is? To experience healing, you've got to first get this answer correct. You can never experience healing until you have discovered the identity of Christ.

> *"He said to them, 'But who do you say that I am?' Simon Peter answered and said, 'You are the Christ, the Son of the living God.'"*
>
> —Matt 16:15–17 NKJV

Jesus did face his identity issue early in his ministry immediately after his baptism with the temptations in the wilderness. He won that war. Now the question is for us to decide.

A PARABLE OF IDENTITY

Second, you must know the identity of what Jesus must take authority over. The Holy Spirit can reveal this. *The Prisoner* was a very popular television series in the sixties, and now is available on DVD and video. In the series, a British secret agent has resigned for unknown reasons and returns home, only to find himself gassed and then waking up on a strange island. The environment seems pleasant and friendly. He has no name on this island, however, and is always referred to as "Number 6." Searching for who or whatever has imprisoned him, he finds a "Number 2," but no "Number 1." This "Number 2" is always calling him "Number 6" and constantly trying to break him down to discover why he resigned. The prisoner replies that he is not a number, saying "I am a free man." Then he asks for "Number 1," a request that is not granted. Everything seems so pleasant his captors wonder why he doesn't accept it and tell them what they want to know.

The series is really a parable of each of us. We are prisoners in a small story created by the Enemy. Our identity has been stolen by this Enemy. Our goal is our freedom, even if it means our death—and it will, eventually. We are imprisoned by our mortal body, the lies of the Enemy, and our lack of belief in the larger story. Like the prisoner, we have lost our identity. The Enemy tries to make things pleasant so that we don't search for the larger story. He doesn't want us to experience the freedom that Christ can give us.

ANOTHER PARABLE OF IDENTITY

In the movie *The Matrix* [1], we see another character struggling with his identity. Tom Anderson in the film is an everyman who goes to work every day and lives in a small story of how he perceives reality. Tom is a computer analyst in what appears to be 1999. In reality, it is over 200 years in the future with the earth as we know it destroyed. The computers with their artificial intelligence have taken over the world, with the humans now no more than biochemical food for the computers. The Matrix is this 1999 projection the computer puts into the minds of the pod-bound humans of this artificially-controlled world to keep them passive and unaware of the reality of the situation. Sure, it's a disturbing story. Unlike most science fiction, you feel you are in the story and can feel Tom's pain. You *are* in the story, more than you know.

Underneath the destroyed world lives a remnant of humanity that somehow escaped the Matrix. Traveling in the sewers of the old city in a high-tech submarine, their destination is Zion, the only place in this world that the humans still control.

From this world of reality a message reaches Tom in the Matrix that he has a purpose and identity, and Tom is given a new name—Neo. With his new name is the message to "Wake Up, Neo. The Matrix has you!" He hears for the first time that he is called to a life of adventure, battle, and risk. Soon Tom stands before Morpheus and a lady known as Trinity in a real world. Morpheus shows Tom two pills—a red one and a blue one. If he takes the blue one, he goes back to La-la land and all this is no more than a dream. Take the red one and he accepts his new identity as Neo and enters into all the authority, adventure, battle, and risk his choice entails. *He has the freedom to make the choice.* Neo takes the red pill.

What happens next is probably the most violent part of the movie. For the first time Neo sees the Matrix for what it is. He sees the millions of humans as nothing more than the biochemical food for the computers, destroyed as they live their false reality. Neo is violently ripping the cables out of his body, cables that suck his own life away from him. Then Morpheus[2] begins the challenging job of discipling Neo for the task he is called to do. You watch as Tom/Neo fails his first test of faith. Over and over in the movie you hear the command given to Tom to wake up.

Some rather violent Agents (software projections in the Matrix) come into Neo's life and try to destroy him. They always call him by his old name, sneering at his thinking he has any authority or strength for what is involved. *The attack is always against his new name.*

Near the end of the story we see the final battle that takes place in a subway station. Our hero is losing the battle with the Agents as they sneer his old name over and over again. Even though near death, Tom continues his fight. Suddenly, instead of running, Tom turns to the Agents and his expression changes.

"I am Neo."

One of the leaders among the remnant watching from the larger (real) world, turns and asks.

"What is he doing?"

Another turns with the answer, "He's beginning to believe."

You then watch as Tom Anderson dies to himself (his vital signs flat-line) and he is reborn as Neo. Trinity reaches to him from the real world and loves this dead body through the rebirth. Look closely at this point and the film image will look very much like the Pieta, the sculpture of Mary holding the body of Christ after the crucifixion. The call from Trinity, again, is to wake up. Neo's new name defines his purpose in life. He awakes as Neo and joins others as the remnant continues to Zion. Now he has purpose—to destroy the Matrix.

In the same way, your new and mythic name defines your purpose in life. It defines why God created you. With it, as with Neo, comes the call to wake up and the take on the new name.

> "It's in Christ that we find out who we are and what we are living for."
>
> —Eph. 1:11 *The Message*

We are all bound and deceived by the Matrix, a virtual world authored by Satan. The Agents in the Matrix story are the demons (spirit guides) sent to accuse us. Each of us is called out of the Matrix to a world of adventure and intimacy with God. We each have the freedom to choose between that blue pill and stay in the deceptive world or take the red pill (the blood of Jesus) and take on the destiny, adventure, battle, and risk that goes with it. Like Tom/Neo, we are called to wake up.

Once we are called out and separated, as with Neo, we are in a war to destroy the Matrix, the Agents, and principalities of that world.

> "Finally, my brethren, be strong in the Lord and in the power of His might. Put on the whole armor of God, that you may be able to stand against the wiles of the devil. For we do not wrestle against flesh and blood, but against principalities, against powers, against the rulers of the darkness of this age, against spiritual hosts of wickedness in the heavenly places."
>
> —Eph 6:10–13 NKJV

Then Paul continues by telling us how to win this war. Notice in Paul's list all the items for the battle are defensive except two.

"Therefore take up the whole armor of God, that you may be able to withstand in the evil day, and having done all, to stand. Stand therefore, having girded your waist with truth, having put on the breastplate of righteousness, and having shod your feet with the preparation of the gospel of peace; above all, taking the shield of faith with which you will be able to quench all the fiery darts of the wicked one. And take the helmet of salvation, and the sword of the Spirit, which is the word of God; praying always with all prayer and supplication in the Spirit, being watchful to this end with all perseverance and supplication for all the saints—."

—Eph 6:13–19 NKJV

The first offensive weapon is the sword of the Spirit, which is the *rhema* of God. Remember, there is no Bible at this time. The Greek word used here indicates that the very speaking of the word has power in it. The *rhema* is a command of God. When God created the world, he spoke it into existence. When Jesus healed someone, he spoke the healing into existence.

The word "power" in this definition is *dunamis,* or the power to do (not the power of control). It really translates as force or miraculous power. The word *dunamis* is the same word used in Luke 9:1 when he sent the disciples out with the *dunamis* and authority to cure diseases and do deliverance.

"Then He called His twelve disciples together and gave them power and authority over all demons, and to cure diseases."

—Luke 9:1 NKJV

The word used for authority here is *exousia,* which translates as freedom, superhuman, and delegated influence.

The second offensive weapon we see in the passage is prayer, for it is from prayer that we find the *rhema* to speak into healing.

DISCOVERING YOUR IDENTITY

The key question, then, is: What is your identity? What is your mythic name? What is your God-given purpose in life? It is through this discovery that we gain the *dunamis* to accomplish what God has called us to do and to experience our personal healing.

The Apostle Paul gives several teachings on this, with a beautiful chapter on spiritual giftings in 1 Corinthians 12. These include not only the gift of healings (notice the plural) but also the gift of wisdom, knowledge, faith, miracle working, prophecy, discernment, and more. In the next chapter, Paul admonishes that the gifts are to be exercised in love. A common aspect of each miracle Christ did was his deep compassion, and Paul says this should be the motivation for using these gifts.

The clue to discovering our identity and purpose was given at the beginning of this chapter. To experience healing, we must pray for God to reveal his purpose (*his* purpose, not ours.). Embracing the purpose will lead us to another identity, destiny, and our mythic name. This type of prayer is called an *identity prayer*. We are asking God to reveal our new name, identity, purpose, and calling. Since this is so important in even our own healing and process, we can always expect God to answer this prayer if we are truly surrendered to him. We should continue this identity prayer until God answers. Use a journal to dialog this journey.

As with Neo, healing begins with taking the "red pill." It begins, as with Neo, with death to self and a rebirthing to the Will of God and destiny for our life. Without that, we can't even see the Matrix and what everything is all about. This is the hardest part, as everything we see and hear tends to contradict this. What does it mean, for example, that the least is the greatest, to give is to receive, to die is to live, to be poor is to be rich, or weakness is strength?

With me, after a few years of struggle someone came to me in a dream and said your spiritual gift is…, and named it. The gift wasn't even in the Apostle Paul's list, but my visitor in the dream was right. Now there is passion in terms of that message. You must struggle with everything you have (even if it means your death) until you hear the message.

EXPRESSING YOUR IDENTITY

There are then three aspects to your personal calling and uniqueness: the passion, the gifts, and the style.

First, you must discover your passion. What really excites you as you live? My pastor's five-year old kid likes to go with him on visits to a retirement home. She literally comes alive as she explores things that the pastor hardly notices. She will sit in front of a lady in a catatonic state, waving her hands in a passionate attempt to bring her out of her lostness. She will dance, sing songs, and embrace the joy of her life. Anything to wake this catatonic woman. Each of us can identify with this catatonic woman. What will it take for God to wake you?

Second, what spiritual gifts does God give to you to bring to the party? The list is much longer that the original list Paul spells out in his epistles. Today there are writing gifts, technical gifts, musical gifts—the list is quite lengthy. The word in the Bible used for healing gifts is plural, implying there are multiple types of healing gifts. I think of blind Ken Medema, who has wonderful music gifts. Ken's most comfortable, however, when using these gifts to heal others. He's not a performer, he's a healer. Most of his music is created during a one-on-one encounter with someone who is hurting as he helps them face their wound by creating with his music.

Finally, what is the style in which you express these gifts? The style for one person with an evangelism gift may be quite different from that of another with this same evangelism gift. We should not judge the other for their style or gifting. God created each of us for the upbuilding of his Church.

THE INCREDIBLE PROPHECY

Most of us are familiar with the incredible prophecy of Jeremiah to his people, which applies to us today as well:

> *"For I know the thoughts that I think toward you, says the LORD, thoughts of peace and not of evil, to give you a future and a hope."*
>
> —Jer. 29:11 NKJV

Unfortunately, we often take this as a type of prosperity gospel and never read the rest of the passage:

> *"For I know the thoughts that I think toward you, says the LORD, thoughts of peace and not of evil, to give you a future and a hope. Then you will call upon Me and go and pray to Me, and I will listen to you. And you will seek Me and find Me..."*
>
> —Jer. 29:11–13a NKJV

You still aren't reading it as it is supposed to be read. These verses refer to a covenant relationship between God and his people; that is, between you and God. What is it that God asks of you? Read the last part of the verse!

> *"Then you will call upon Me and go and pray to Me, and I will listen to you. And you will seek Me and find Me, when you search for Me with* **all** *your heart."*
>
> —Jer. 29:12–13 NKJV, emphasis added

We tend to leave out the *all* word. God requires us to seek his face with our *all* our heart. Now, what does God promise? One thing, of course, is that we will find him. Look at the rest of what he promises:

> *I will be found by you, says the LORD, and I will bring you back from your captivity; I will gather you from all the nations and from all the places where I have driven you, says the LORD, and*

I will bring you to the place from which I cause you to be carried away captive.

—Jer. 29:14 NKJV

Here God promises two more things:

1. He will release us from captivity.

2. He will restore place

Some time ago a friend and I lunched with someone who felt they were in captivity. My friend and I were the only contacts this person had with anything spiritual (this person could verbalize this to us). This person said they had no *place*. As a child with family this person had place. I showed this verse and the promise. *All this person had to do was seek the face of God with their* **whole** *heart, and God would honor that and they would find him and a new name, be released from captivity, and find place again!*

Is your city in captivity? Is your church in captivity? Are you in captivity? What does God promise? What do you have to do to claim the promise?

A few months ago I spent two days alone at the beach, seeking the face of God (or, as I told my pastor, "getting face time with the Boss"). There in the quiet room I was reading a chapter in a book by Dutch Sheets on listening to God. As I read story after story in the chapter, I suddenly became aware of a horn that sounded in the distance every few seconds (not minutes, seconds).

The horn had been going all morning, but I was just now hearing it for the first time. I fell to my knees before God, realizing he been speaking to me all morning, and yet now I was hearing him for the first time.

The horn is on a buoy, and works from the wind that blows through it. It warns approaching ships of danger. How like that, God is often trying to warn us of danger, yet we aren't listening.

When I shared this story later with a pastor, he told me there was more to the message God was giving me. The Captain of a ship has to be able to hear the horn in the noise of the storm in the darkness of the night. He does this by learning to hear the horn in the quietness of the day. Once he has learned what the horn sounds like, it is much easier for him to hear the horn in the storm at night. How like our intimacy with God! We must first learn to hear him in the quietness of the day, and then we can hear him in the storms of life. Remember the story of Peter recognizing Jesus in the storm? The reason Peter could recognize the voice of Jesus in the storm is that he had learned to hear Jesus in the quiet of the day.

YOU CAN HAVE THE NEW NAME NOW

In Revelation the Apostle John speaks of a white stone God gives us when we arrive in Heaven before him.

> *"He who has an ear, let him hear what the Spirit says to the churches. To him who overcomes I will give some of the hidden manna to eat. And I will give him a white stone, and on the stone a new name written which no one knows except him who receives it."*
>
> —Rev 2:17 NKJV

On this stone is a secret name that is known only to him. At this point God reveals that secret name (identity, mythic name) to us, and there is healing and restoration. There is intimacy with God, *total* healing, and restoration. That is what Heaven is all about. We are back in the Garden, we are back with a rich intimacy with God. There is complete healing. Sharing my journey with a lady a few weeks ago, I told her this story. Her reply was astounding:

"Carl, you can have that white stone now."

She was right. What is binding you, keeping you from seeing and taking that white stone and the new name?

THE FINAL HEALING AND THE RESULT

Now let's return to the story of the demoniac and apply this. The second time Jesus reached out to heal him he asked the man what was his name (identity). The man is mute, and it is the demonic spirits that reply.

"My name is Legion, for we are many."

Doesn't even sound grammatically correct, does it? A Legion was a regiment of 6000 Roman soldiers. There were 6000 territorial demonic spirits in control of this man. No wonder he was wild! They were pulling in 6000 different directions, confusing him. In the Luke version, we see the demonic spirits asking Jesus not to be thrown into the abyss. They knew the endgame; that is, how the story would end eventually in time. That's the way most people play the game. They know the endgame, they just don't change. In the other gospels the demonic spirits beg Jesus to put them in the pigs. In that way, they would remain in the territory (remember, they are territorial spirits). They knew Jesus was going to take authority and they could no longer live in the man.

Jesus does take authority, heals the man, and the demonic spirits are sent to the pigs. There are about 2000 pigs here, together worth about $250,000 (that's a quote from Barclay using 1960 values). They all rush screaming over a high cliff and into the water. Jesus is tricky—he did what they wanted, but then the pigs rushed over the cliff and were drowned in the water. If you do spiritual mapping, water is often a territorial boundary. Jesus caused the territorial spirits to leave the territory and they were gone. (When I shared this with my pastor, he made an interesting comment. He'd done a lot of research on this, he told me, and this is the first example of deviled ham in the Bible.)

The swine herders, seeing this, rushed into the village. The people of the village then rushed out to see things. There was the "wild" man now healed and sitting calmly and clothed. Then Mark tells us something very interesting—they were afraid. They pleaded with Jesus to leave the area. The man's identity, however, was changed. Now he is "the man who has been healed by Jesus."

THE REACTION

"A rhino can run thirty miles an hour. A rhino, however, can only see thirty feet ahead. What's at thirty-one feet, however, doesn't make any difference.

—Erwin McManus

Look closely at the result by the village. Why did they ask Jesus to leave the area? Why were they afraid? What Jesus did and said was very threatening to the people there. Their comfort zone was disturbed. We want Jesus near us. We want to hear his words. We want the healing that he gives. At the same time, however, we hold a sense of anxiety about what he will demand of us. The price is high.

Remember this is a cross-cultural journey for Jesus. This is a Greek culture. Jesus stands for the moment outside of their culture. The man who is healed, however, is a part of their culture. We don't know if he was Greek or not, but he could reach their culture. Soon we will see Jesus sending him into the culture.

In the story of the demoniac, where are you in the story? Are you the demoniac, fractured and broken? A disciple, silent (bound by fear) but seeking and scared? The crowd, bound by fear about a possible change?

WHY DESTROY THE PIGS?

There is a question here that is important. Why did Jesus have to destroy 2000 pigs to heal the man? The man believed he was bound by the demonic spirits, and lived into that belief. His belief shaped his behavior. Both Mark and Luke say the man was shouting and shrieking. To destroy this belief, he and those watching needed a visible demonstration It is now the pigs that are shrieking and shouting, and the pigs rush to the water, are destroyed, and the area is suddenly very quiet. Very quiet. The man now believes he is healed by Jesus (and he is), and his behavior follows this new belief.

In the same way, our behavior follows our belief. Whether the belief is right or wrong, we act from the visions we hold. We can choose to have a healing vision given to us by Jesus, or choose a fractured life from broken visions.

Dialog

1. What name do you see on your white stone? What is your mythic name?

2. What does that mean to you?

3. Share this name with friends. What do they say about this name?

4. What does the sentence "I have found Place" mean to you?

Notes

1. Before viewing *The Matrix* film, I should give you a warning. This is an R rated film. The story is dark and does have violence in it. It is not the gospel according to Larry and Andy, and Keanu Reeves is not a Messiah. It is a new type of story that defines a new type of myth. The comments here refer only to the first film. It is a secular film, and embraces what *Time* magazine calls a liberal humanism. More accurately, it is a liberal secular humanism, the same religion taught in most of our schools. It also is a parable of postmodern Christianity. The film was scripted by two brothers who know a lot about the Bible, Shakespeare, Greek mythology, Buddhism,

Hinduism, and more. A local pastor preached an excellent 4-part sermon on this film. You can order this pastor's series on tape for $16 by calling 1-800-234-0072. A very good book available on the film is *The Gospel Reloaded*, by Chris Seay (a Houston pastor) and Greg Garrett (a teacher at Baylor University). The extreme popularity of the first film indicates there is a deep spiritual hunger for purpose and meaning on the part of our younger generation, and it is the Church's responsibility to give them the true message.

2. *Morpheus* is the Greek word for *change*. *Matrix* is a Greek word for the womb.

3. It is from Trinity (the woman) that Neo gets his birthing experience. It is from Morpheus (the man) that Neo gets the message he has the strength to destroy the Matrix. This relationship is also true in your life.

8

The Purpose of Healing

"The absolute goal of ministry is to glorify God."

Once the man is healed, he wants to go with Jesus, leaving the darkness and chaos of the area behind him. Jesus, however, gives him a really simple command. Jesus tells him to go back home, *back into the chaos,* and tell his friends what Jesus has done for him. And the Bible says he went throughout the region telling people what Jesus had done for him. This is in Mark 5. The healing is done, but Jesus is forced to leave the area. The man who returns to his home was probably a Gentile.

Now move forward to Mark 7:31 and read what happens there. Jesus returns to the Decapolis area. This time no one is asking him to leave. Jesus heals a deaf man and releases him from a speech impediment. The strategy is different, but the man is healed. Jesus is welcomed.

The remarkable thing here is that the entire region has been transformed from the ministry of one man. All this man had to do was first to be obedient, and then to tell his story. Jesus didn't give him the four spiritual laws (not that anything is wrong with them) or a seminary course in evangelism on how to defend his faith. All he had to do was step into the chaos and tell his story. No one could deny the truth of his story.

LOOKING AT THE BIGGER STORY

This seems like a simple story. In reality, what Jesus did here had tremendous impact on the course of history. Here are a few leaders who emerged from the Decapolis area:

• Philodemus, the great Epicurean philosopher

• Theodorus, the rhetorician who was the tutor of Tiberius, the reigning Roman Emperor

• Menippus, the famous satirist

• Meleager, the master of the Greek epigram

All of these men came from Gadaria area. When this one man obeyed Jesus and returned to the chaos, he was the first missionary to the Greek people group.

Many times we feel overwhelmed and inadequate for what God is calling us to do. To quote Phillip Brooks, you never become truly spiritual by sitting down and wishing to become so. You must undertake something so great that you cannot accomplish it unaided.

Reminds me of the story from the Church of the Saviour in Washington, D.C. When told in 1960 that the site at which they planned to open a coffeehouse had previously been the site for three restaurants that had failed, they simply said "Good. If it succeeds we will know it is not our own doing." The coffeehouse is still there.

THE MYTHS

There are several myths here Jesus moves against. First, there is the myth that one person can't transform a city or even a region. There is just enough truth in this for us to buy it. One person can't, that's true, but one person with God can. In this story we see one person, with God, transformed a region. This still goes on today. In the Transformations I tape from The Sentinel Group,[1] you can see the story of the transformation of four cities. In Transformations II, you can watch the transformation of three regions. Most of these were led by only one or two people who were committed to seeing the Kingdom come.

The second myth is that you can't tell your story until you are well. If that were true, we'd all be waiting. God seems to let each of us have something short of what we expect (such as Paul's thorn in the flesh) to keep us humble and dependent upon the gifts of others in the Church. This makes us need the gifts of others to experience the fullness of our own ministry. That's why we have the Church. Just like in a wonderful marriage, the whole is more than the sum of the parts. The Church brings us together in love, binding our gifts to accomplish together with God what we could not do alone.

The third myth is that there is no spiritual hunger today. Some researchers have reported that my state, Oregon, is one of the most unchurched states in the country. A secular survey of the Portland area, however, showed that in Portland one of the *primary* needs of the city was that of an unmet spiritual hunger. What a challenge for the local church!

INTO THE CHAOS

What is the Decapolis, or chaos, God is asking you to step into? Jesus asked the man to go back to the chaos and tell his story. We often assume it is "out there," whether Seattle, the slums of our city, an undeveloped country, or wherever. It is, however, more likely within. This is where this demoniac was at the beginning of the story with his chaos within. Jesus first met that chaos. Now the man has authority to move beyond that to the chaos of his community.

You might ask why moving in the chaos is so important. Isn't the man already healed? The answer to this lies in the purpose of the healing. Why did Jesus heal him in the first place? The purpose of the healing was to glorify God. The second purpose of healings, which we see in Acts, is to build up the Church (see the story in Acts 3–4). It has nothing to do with our agenda, and everything to do with God's agenda. We really don't know this man's given name, the given name of the man by the Pool of Bethesda, or the given name of the lame man in Acts 3. Although names are very important, our true names represent an identity that God has for us.

I remember some time ago coming out of a restaurant and holding the door open for a young lady in a wheelchair. Since I lived in a wheelchair for six months in 1989, something happens to me inside when I see someone in a wheelchair. It is a deep pain that sears across my heart. I wanted to tell her to stand up, to take authority in God's name for healing, and for her to run again. As I held the door, she started thanking me. Once outside, she continued to thank me as I turned a different direction and walked to my car. I was feeling guilty that I hadn't asked her to stand up. What if she hadn't been able to stand up? I would have looked like a fool. As I continued to my car, God spoke very clearly to me.

"All I wanted you to do, Carl, was to tell her your story. I will do the rest. You have no authority. I have all authority."

Now I really felt guilty! I hadn't even done that. In the telling of the story we glorify God and cut through the bindings of the heart.

THE PURPOSE

In the healing of the lame man by the pool, the release of the demoniac, the raising of Lazarus, the healing of the Samaritan woman (and the rest of a long list) Jesus always had two purposes. The first was to glorify God, and the second was to bring unity. That is the purpose of the Church, as the Body of Christ, today.

THE WARNING

Once we have discovered our identity and purpose we begin to take on our mythic name and to live at a very dangerous place. At this point the Enemy knows we have power and authority and will do anything to destroy us. His primary target is always our heart.

The Enemy will first try to make us believe he isn't there and there is no war going on. If we buy this, he's home free, but our heart is still bound. If we get beyond this and embrace the war, he will try to discourage us. He will strike at relationships. He will try to destroy the unity (Chapter 13). He aims at the marriage, church, anything to break the unity. He will try to make us believe we lack the authority and power for the battle.

The stories of my own battle with the virus and the story of the loss of my wife are vivid examples of this. The Enemy always strikes for the heart. If the heart is wounded, all else is gone.

"To live in ignorance of spiritual warfare is the most naïve and dangerous thing a person can do. It's like skipping through the worst part of town, late at night, waving your wallet above your head. It's like walking into an al-Qaida training camp, wearing an 'I love the United States' T-shirt...And let me tell you something: you don't escape spiritual warfare simply because you choose not to believe it exists or because you refuse to fight it. The bottom line is, you are going to have to fight for your heart."

—John Eldredge, *Waking the Dead: The Glory of a Heart Fully Alive* [2]

Be very sure you know your purpose and identity, that you stay focused, and that you are on God's agenda. I enjoy reading one of the Psalms every day. Over and over again in these psalms you see a consistent pattern. David is under relentless pursuit from Saul, who is determined to kill him. Sometimes, David says, his house is surrounded and there seems no escape. Each time, however, you see a consistent message as he reaches the end of his song—he is praising God for saving him. The most classic of these, of course, is Psalms 23 that ends with a banquet table before him and oil, a symbol of both healing and authority, poured on his head.

Dialog

1. Why do you think Jesus didn't stay in the area?

2. Where is your real Decapolis? Within or Without? Both?

3. Can you risk going into it?

Notes

1. Both tapes are available from the Sentinel Group, P.O Box 6334, Lynnwood, WA 98036. You can also order toll-free at 1–800–668–5657. Their website is http://www.sentinelgroup.org.

2. Eldredge, John. *Waking the Dead: The Glory of a Heart Fully Alive.* (Thomas Nelson Publishers: Nashville) 2003, p. 152

9

The Wilderness and Healing

"Healing is not an issue of faith, but rather an affair of the heart. If the romance and passion is there in the heart, we will have faith."

"We each face our own wilderness in our healing. The way out is often as close as that tree at the springs of Marah. The way out depends on hearing God. Hearing God depends on us having intimacy with him. Wilderness decisions are often life and death. In the wilderness God can do things he can do no other place. In the wilderness, it is easy to pray dangerous prayers. Often the wilderness is the safest place to be."

When we find ourselves in the wilderness and aching for the healing, there is a great sense of frustration. Jesus wants us healed, yet there we are without the healing. Pastor Ron Mehl here in Portland (author of *God Works the Night Shift* and other books) constantly fought a long battle with leukemia and recently the Lord took him home. At the same time he was fighting this, the church he pastored grew from about two dozen to over six thousand. He also wrote many books on healing. People from many other churches sat under his teaching at times and prayed for his healing. You can probably name others who physically or emotionally remain broken in some way, yet you can sense the healing they have experienced when you are with them and they bring healing to you.

WILDERNESS EXPERIENCES OF THE BIBLE

Let's first look at some examples of wilderness experiences in the Bible and how the "hero" acted. At first impression, we might say the Bible begins and ends with a Garden. This, however, is not as true as you might think. The Bible begins and ends with a wilderness.

The First Wilderness

When Adam was created, he was created in the wilderness. The Garden of Eden did not exist at his creation. There, in the wilderness, he had intimacy with God. The wilderness was Place. Place is where there is intimacy with God. Later God created woman and the Garden of Eden and placed Adam and Eve in the Garden. They still had their intimacy with God. There was a healing and eternal life through this intimacy. There was no sickness.

Then Adam and Eve sinned, and Man lost his intimacy with God. As a result we live in a broken world. God had given Man authority and stewardship of the earth, and the Enemy stole the authority from Man as well as taking, through Man, authority of the earth. Christ came to give us a path to that intimacy again. He became Man, and through his death made our healing possible. In the Model Prayer that Christ gave us, we pray for his will on earth as it (already) is in heaven.

The Wilderness of Jacob

In the story of Jacob in Genesis 28, we see that Jacob was sent away from his home by his father (Isaac) to find a wife. More likely, Isaac was trying to save Jacob's life after he had stolen the birthright from his brother. Jacob was in both a geographic and personal wilderness with no Place. Jacob had departed from Beersheba and was traveling toward Haran.

The scriptures than say;

"So he came to a certain place and stayed there all night, because the sun had set."

—Gen 28:11 NKJV

You can then read the story of Jacob's fantastic dream while he is in this wilderness—the ladder descending from heaven to that place and the angels coming up and down the ladder. When Jacob awakes, he has experienced a remarkable healing. The place (geographic and personal) he assumed was wilderness was actually Place, a place of intimacy with God. Jacob builds an altar.

In the Hebrew, the word used for "came to" in this story is *paga*. This is the first time this Hebrew word is used in the Bible. In our language, the closest meaning we can get to the word in a secular sense is serendipity, or "accidental" discovery.[1] What Jacob suddenly "chanced upon" was a Place, or a place in his own life of intimacy with God. Within this Place he could pray anything and God would answer, because God's will became his will. It is the same with us, at *paga* place, you can pray anything and God will answer because your will becomes God's will.

Another Greek word is related here—*karios,* or a window God gives us in time where we can act. If we fail to act in this window, the moment may never come again. When the Israelites first reached the land of Canaan, this was a *karios* moment in time. They could choose to go in, or turn back. God had already given them the land. God's orders were to take it. They failed, and an entire generation except for two died in the wilderness. It's a simple equation:

Paga + *karios*-> God's Place and healing

A more correct version of the passage is:

When Jacob came to The Place...

This *paga* place becomes God's Place in the wilderness. A place of accidental discovery. A place of intercessory prayer. Jacob renamed the place Bethel, which means House of God, a place built for the presence of God to dwell.

What does this say about the word *paga*? In the spiritual sense, Dutch Sheets[2] says it is another word for intercession. We don't have enough wisdom to pray correctly. We "chance upon" the words to say in prayer, and the prayer takes us to God's Place. Dutch says in teaching this in one class a student informed him that this is the word in Israel that is used in target shooting when one hits the bull's eye. The Hebrew translation says he or she has hit the *paga*. Isn't that like our prayer? In *paga* prayer, we hit the bull's eye! Paga Places, like Jacob's dream, take us to the very Gates of Heaven!

The Wilderness of Moses

Moses had a rich life in Egypt growing up in the House of Pharaoh. He would have the best education, high standard of living, rich food, and the good life. He kills an Egyptian in anger, then is banished to the wilderness with only a rod and a staff. No car, no computer, no wife. He is only 40 years old. Just the rod and staff. In the wilderness, the rod is used for protection. A shepherd would use it to fight a wild animal in protecting the sheep. The staff was a symbol of support.

> *"Your rod and Your staff, they comfort me"*
>
> —Psalm 23:4b NKJV

Look at the full verse:

> *Yea, though I walk through the valley of the shadow of death,*
> *I will fear no evil;*
> *For You are with me;*
> *Your rod and Your staff, they comfort me.*
>
> —Psalm 23:4 NKJV

Like Moses or David, when we find ourselves in the wilderness, there is still that rod and that staff and the Presence of God. Probably unknown to Moses, he was beginning a 40-year seminary course in wilderness survival training. How would you like to take a 40-year course before beginning as a pastor, missionary, teaching job, or whatever?

Now move forward in time forty years as God tells Moses he has a job for him. Moses is going to need that rod to get the Israelites out of Egypt and through the wilderness. Can you see how preposterous that is from our human view? What is the rod that God has given you to get his people out of their binding?

Moses met God in the wilderness at the burning bush after forty years in the wilderness.

Again we see *paga*, a place of accidental discovery. Moses meets God at *paga*, and the *paga* place in the wilderness becomes a God's Place. Moses was eighty years old as he returned to Egypt to take on this ministry.

The Israelites left Egypt with Moses and now we see them reaching the waters of Marah.

> *"Now when they came to Marah, they could not drink the waters*
> *of Marah, for they were bitter…"*
>
> —Exodus 15:23

A desert traveler knows you can only go about three days without water. The Israelites had traveled three days and had no water. They would have been close to death as they reach the oasis of Marah. Falling on their faces at the water, they started drinking quickly—only to discover the water was bitter. Now they would surely die. Their stomachs experienced very severe cramps in a few minutes.

Here at the very beginning of their wilderness journey Moses used his wilderness training and was beginning to understand what God was doing. Jamie Buckingham (in his *A Way Through the Wilderness*) tells us those bitter springs are still there. The water will be oily to the touch. You can put your hand in the water and feel the water (don't lick the fingers).

The reason the water was bitter and felt oily at these springs is that the water in these springs had a high content of magnesium and calcium. It would be like someone dehydrated and near death drinking milk of magnesia. Moses cried to the Lord. God directed Moses to a nearby tree. Moses broke the limbs to release the sap, and then put the wood in the water. This initiated a chemical reaction that caused the magnesium to precipitate to the bottom, leaving the water sweet. Now they could drink. The "tree" that Moses put in the water symbolized the cross, which later would be cast into our own bitter waters.

Buckingham tells us there was also a second aspect of the springs of Marah. The Israelites were used to the rich food of the Egyptians. Now they would be eating manna. The Israelites' stomachs had to be purged, preparing the digestive systems for the manna of the wilderness.

God was *testing* the Israelites. It wasn't so much a knowledge test (quoting Jamie Buckingham), but rather a test of whether they could listen and obey. Without the rich Egyptian food, they would actually be healthier.

> "...I will put none of the diseases on you which I have brought on the Egyptians, For I am the Lord who heals you."
>
> —Exodus 15:26b

This was a conditional statement. Read the first part of the verse!

> "If you diligently heed the voice of the LORD your God and do what is right in His sight, give ear to His commandments and keep all His statutes, I will put none of the diseases on you which I have brought on the Egyptians. For I am the LORD who heals you."
>
> —Exodus 15:26

Read carefully the wilderness story of Moses, as the exodus is a story of each of us. Moses is a foreshadowing of Christ, and is prophet, priest, judge, lawgiver, intercessor, victor, exile, fugitive, guide, shepherd, healer, and miracle-worker. Just as Christ births our freedom, it is through Moses that the freedom of the Israelites was birthed. The stick in the springs was a symbol of the cross cast in our own bitter waters. The Ten Commandments fell broken as a symbol of our own failure to keep them. The serpent on the cross that brought healing to the Israelites was a foreshadowing of the Cross of Christ. Twice Moses faced the challenge of getting water from a rock. The first time he was told to strike the rock (symbolizing the striking of Christ before the crucifixion). The second time God told him only to speak to the rock, as in striking the rock he would be crucifying Christ again.

> *"...and all drank the same spiritual drink. For they drank of that spiritual Rock that followed them, and that Rock was Christ."*
>
> —1 Cor 10:4 NKJV

Moses failed this second time, striking the rock. As a result, he could not enter the Promised Land. The Israelites eventually stood out of the wilderness and on the edge of the Promised Land (or "time"). They, like us, (and Elisha's servant, blind Bartimaeus) could not see. But Moses did see. In Numbers 14 he claims the vision he sees and in so doing moves the hand of God and saves the nation.

We each face our own wilderness in our healing. The way out is often as close as that tree by the springs. The way out depends on hearing God. Hearing God depends on us having intimacy with him. Wilderness decisions are often life and death. In the wilderness God can do things he can do no other place. In the wilderness, it is easy to pray dangerous prayers. Often the wilderness is the safest place to be. There eventually comes a time, however, when God tells us to take the risk of moving out of our wilderness, just as with the Israelites.

The Wildernesses of the New Testament

In the New Testament we see almost every spiritual leader turning to the wilderness before their ministry. John the Baptist always looked like he had just come from the wilderness. Jesus began his ministry in the wilderness. The Apostle Paul went to the desert after his conversion. Why did these men to this?

I've tried my own wilderness experience in the mountains of Virginia. The experience is not one you can put in the English language. Every word spoken to you in the wilderness becomes like the finest gold and pierces the heart. Every sense is quickened to a level you never have experienced before. What happens is beyond any drug you could take and doesn't cost a dime—but it could cost you everything you own. It takes you to God's Place—*paga*, and that's a very incredible place to be.

The Last Wilderness

The New Testament (and the Bible) ends with another wilderness story. John has been banished to the island of Patmos, a wilderness and an experience of deep loneliness for a man who loved people, relationships, and the early church. John, over 90 years old, is such a threat to the established order that the Roman Empire shipped him to this island. Legends say they tried to burn him in oil; but even that didn't kill him. So there he is, isolated from the church and the people he loved and alone in the wilderness of Patmos. The island is about six miles from north to south, and about ten miles wide at its widest point. It was a traditional place of banishment for political prisoners. And what happens? He has this incredible vision of Heaven that he recorded for us. This vision is so incredible that he can't communicate in any kind of language he knew of, so he used symbols. The symbols are rich, difficult to understand. Many of the symbols are particularly meaningful in the culture of that time, but some of the cultural significance is lost with time.

WHAT WILDERNESS ARE YOU TRAVELING IN?

In 1989 when I was suddenly paralyzed from the shoulders down, the first reaction was that I had entered a real wilderness. Doctors said I would never walk again. Income was shut down. There were bills to pay. This didn't look like it would be any fun. As I lay there on the bed with my wife at my side, I turned to her and made a bold statement.

"We are starting out on one big adventure!"

I was thrashing about on the bed with the therapists, trying to get them to start working on getting my legs back. I desperately wanted those legs working again. The therapists were doing these stupid exercises asking me to bring my arm down at a diagonal across my chest against their resistance. As a Type A personality, this limitation was very frustrating. Finally, one therapist told me what they were doing.

"Carl, you can't move enough oxygen through your lungs for us to start on the legs. The lungs are very weak, and we have to build the lungs up some before starting any work on the legs." It would be many months before I could leave a wheelchair, and at this point I didn't have the strength to move to a wheelchair.

Then God started speaking to me.

"Hey Carl! It's like your spiritual journey. You thrash around trying to do things, but you don't have enough of the wind of the Holy Spirit yet to do what I want you to do. You have to build up those spiritual lungs first."

During those months of wilderness God spoke often. He was trying to teach me to lay still and listen. I also learned volumes about my neural system, my muscles, respiratory system, and physical limitations at any given time. Soon I was going into online medical databases finding out more information on the virus that had attacked my body, what it had done to the neural system (it had destroyed the nerves), whether it could be rebuilt (it couldn't), and much more. I felt that the healing when it came (and it did) would have to be from God.

The wilderness became an adventure. It was where I was supposed to be at that time. It was preparation for a greater ministry. God was doing something there He could do no other place. I could walk with God safely.

Healing is not an issue of faith, but rather an affair of the heart. If the romance and passion is there in the heart, we will have faith.

I've gone to the wilderness here in Oregon. I expected it to be dead—no life. What surprised me was that, for those who wish to see, there *is* life there. Only you have to look for it. I found plants and animals I had never seen before.

What is the wilderness and rod that God has given you to get His people out of their binding?

Dialog

1. What is your wilderness?

2. How do you feel about it?

3. Is there life in this wilderness?

4. What is your rod? What is the difference between a rod and a staff?

Notes

1. I really don't like the word "accidental." I very seldom use it in conversation. It implies something is happening that is outside of God's agenda. I use it several times in this chapter because there is no English equivalent. It looks accidental to us, but is really part of a plan we have yet to understand.

2. Sheets, Dutch. *Intercessory Prayer: How God Can Use Your Prayers to Move Heaven and Earth.* (Revel: Ventura, CA) 1996. pp. 98–101

10

The Wounded Healer:
Leadership Issues

"The mantle from those who mentor us often falls on us. Choose your mentors carefully."

Some years ago I worked with a ministry team that met weekly for ministry. One lady always showed up with alcohol on her breath, something I thought was not the best approach to ministry. We had a business meeting for planning, and she brought her own bottle with her on those evenings, sharing it with others in the group. I didn't drink, and soon I was the only one not drinking.

I called the pastor of the church, sharing that I considered the group had a problem and wished to discuss this with him. He agreed, and at a church supper a few days later I shared a table with just him and his wife. I shared the drinking problem of the group, and then mentioned to him that I had a problem with this and felt it separated me from the unity of our ministry. Since the unity we shared was the primary witness we had in the world, I felt this lack of unity was hurting our ministry and witness to the larger world.

The pastor agreed that I had a problem, and told me the first step would be to share with the community that I had a problem. I mentally made a note of this. He asked me if I could do this, and I told him I could. He was holding me accountable for taking this first step.

After this, I waited to hear the second step. He never gave me any second step. He soon turned to a man at a nearby table and began talking with him. I only had the one step, and I had committed myself to doing it.

It took me about two weeks to get up the courage to share this with the group. We had a prayer and sharing time before each ministry session, but it took a little time to get the courage. Finally I shared. Confessing to the group, I said that I was having a problem with the drinking (and also added the smoking) of the group and that it separated me from the rest of the group, and how this was hurting the unity of our witness.

"Yes," they said, "we agree you have a problem. We will pray with you about that problem."

In a few minutes we went from worship to ministry. Nothing had changed. I wrestled with this a few more weeks, praying to God to give me answers and what I should do next, as well as exploring my own feelings about the issue and their response.

A few weeks later the group leader shared with us from a meeting with the pastor. It seems a young man had come into the church with a serious drinking problem. His family was broken, he had lost his job, there was a major depression, and this only led him to more drinking. The pastor wondered if it would be permissible to put this man in our ministry group and maybe we could help him.

We all agreed, and soon he was an integral part of the group. The alcohol problem vanished overnight and was never an issue again.

Now this story has an interesting point. This man who was lonely, depressed, broken, alcoholic, and apparently lost to any reality gave a gift to the group—a true sense of unity—that none of us could give to the group. His woundedness was a gift to community that was needed more than anything else. He was a leader to us in terms of this gift. This is always true in the church. We are a leader in terms of our gift, and a follower in terms of the gifts of others. When we experience a deep wounding, it often places us in a leadership position that is not of our choosing. Sure, God is crying because we are trapped in a net that was created years ago with the fall of Adam and Eve. Yet this same God has created a way out through the death and Resurrection of Christ and endows us with spiritual gifts beyond our capacity to understand.

When I visit someone in the hospital, I make the assumption they are the wounded one and I'm there to cheer them up. Frequently, though, I find this person, from their wilderness, speaks into my life with words of healing. The room becomes *paga*. As the old saying goes, we are all beggars looking for bread.

LEADERSHIP, HEALING, AND GIFTS

Years later I went through another leadership experience. I had lost my wife after a battle with leukemia, and there was still a deep loneliness and depression from this. She had been an incredible woman, and what had happened made absolutely no sense at all. Soon the elders asked me to be the lead elder, which I really wrestled with and accepted after three days of prayer, weeping, and fasting. The church was caught up in deep spiritual warfare, and with my own woundedness I personally felt it was no place for me. Yet there was deep trust and a strong faith from me, and the church wanted that. A few months later the pastor resigned, and a few weeks later I stood in the pulpit to give a message. There was a lot of infighting for leadership, soon there would be a false prophet coming in from outside, and we had a deep concern we were losing the church.

My message was simple. If there was to be any leadership, it must be from the gifts of the members. Then, afterwards, I sat at the altar and wept, realizing I had to show them how to do this, and I really didn't know what gifts I brought to the party.

What I didn't know was that that afternoon a pastor from the east was driving through Portland on the way through our city to his in-laws further west. As he passed on the Interstate within two miles of our church (which he probably had never heard of) the Holy Spirit bid him to turn aside and drive to our church property, which was now vacant after the service. There, on the grounds, he knelt in prayer for the church. Exactly one year later he stood in the pulpit as our new pastor and he shared this story with us for the first time.

During this time we were without a pastor God did give extraordinary gifts. There were times when I found I could touch someone and they would be instantly healed. Another time a family was evicted from their apartment and the elders did a prayer march on the apartment and the eviction notice was canceled (with no other steps taken) in less than 24 hours. Another time the elders got a call about a teenager in the hospital with a high fever which was racing higher. The doctors could not control it, and had a grave concern the heart would be damaged. The elders visited, prayed, and 25 minutes after we left the fever abated. I did, however, notice an interesting aspect of the pattern. If at any time I felt I was the hero in this, my gifting would suddenly disappear as if it never existed. God was trying, desperately, to save the church while keeping me humble. Moreover, nothing was being given for my sake or the sake of the person being healed. Each healing was there for the healing of the church and to glorify God.

WHAT IS AUTHENTIC LEADERSHIP?

Dan Webster is head of a Christian organization that trains leaders. He likes to use the illustration of a sailboat story, and tells us that with a sailboat there is a very heavy ballast below the waterline that keeps the sailboat upright. If the boat loses this ballast, it's going to tip over in the slightest storm. With most leadership, all you see is the part above the water. A manager at work can do everything exactly right and succeed in his job, but if things aren't right below the surface, he's going to eventually have problems. A pastor, for example, may preach well, counsel well, and manage his church well. However, today we are finding many pastors with major depressions, moral issues, and other bindings that prevent them from ever reaching their full potential to which God has called them.

As part of his research, Dan interviewed the leaders of other organizations that train leaders and asked them if they saw anything in common among the organizations that consistently showed high growth and high return on the stock market. The leaders who succeeded the best, he discovered, were not the ones with high charisma (in the secular sense) or incredible management talents; but rather all of them shared two common characteristics. First, they had an unerring and passionate commitment to their goals. Second, they were very humble. I could add a third. They are all servant leaders. I like the advertisements for JetBlue airlines, an airline growing dramatically even in the airline slump. There is David Neeleman, the CEO, loading the baggage and cleaning the airplanes. He seems to take great joy in doing any type of servant role with the airline.

This is no surprise to those of us who have studied the life of Christ. Christ himself had an unerring and passionate commitment to his goals. Second, Christ had an incredible sense of humility and mercy. And third, Christ was a servant leader.

THE SERVANT LEADER

A few months ago I had a very interesting dream. Walking down the street, there suddenly appeared in the sky a message directly from God as to what I was supposed to do that day. I thought this was amazing and watched as the message slowly faded. I picked up a newspaper (in the dream), and there in the headlines was a message directly from God as to what I was supposed to do that day. Then the message faded. In each case, the message faded before I could show it or point it out to anyone else. Obviously, God was giving me a personal message about the day.

As I began my morning devotional, I thanked God for the dream and asked him why he couldn't really do that with me. It would greatly help me in planning my day and simplify things.

God replied, "I did. I sent my Son, my only Son. What more do you want me to do?"

Christ embodied the true servant leadership style for us today. It is from our own pain at seeing the darkness from the Enemy's entrance into our world that we experience the gifting necessary to move beyond it. Our woundedness puts us at some special place where we can experience new gifts, passions, and humility. It is a place we would never choose for ourselves.

THE FIRST STEP

What mentor in your life embodies the true leadership style that you see in Christ? This may be an active leader who is mentoring in you now, or perhaps a passive leader who has only spoken in a workshop or whose books you have read. Maybe it was someone in your past, who is now gone on to be with the Lord. They were, however instrumental in being a watershed in your life. How can you live into that leadership style?

If I had to name a key person in my life that fit this description, it would certainly be Howard Rees. I was just out of college and was going into the real world, living and working in the Washington, D.C. area. I was a Type A person, ready to change the world. Just point me in the right direction. Howard Rees always had that incredible smile from the wonderful joy he found in his Christian life. His job was directing the college student programs for the D.C. area, with funding from at least two denominations. He walked with a cane. His legs, I was told, were nothing more than calcified powder that would shatter if he ever fell. Tapping along with his cane, he would always ask these embarrassing questions, like "Where is God working in your life?" That one question, spoken from him one time, led me to one of the most spiritual times I have ever experienced—the journey with a coffee house church At his home, he had a reproduction of Rembrandt's *The Apostle Paul* hanging over his fireplace and mantle. Someone had gotten a copy from the National Gallery of Art in Washington, D.C. (copies are no longer available there) and photographically dropped it to canvas. The canvas was then treated in some way and then baked in an oven to give it the three-dimensional quality of the original.

One day I tried to reach him, only to find he had gone to Switzerland (to find Paul Tournier) and then gone on to Israel. He was in Israel when the six-day war broke out. When he returned home I tried to reach him, only to find he had loaded a car (or maybe cars) with a group of students, some of them African-American, and they were going to crash segregated restaurants while traveling down to North Carolina on the way to a Christian conference for students. The third time I called (and this was all within a few weeks) he had left for the Midwest to see his son graduate from college.

More often, Howard Rees would call me. It might go like this:

"Hey, Carl. Some of the students are meeting over at Paul Geren's house tonight to talk with him. Want to come?"

I didn't know Paul Geren, but it was Rees' invitation. Better go. Now Paul Geren was a Ph.D. from Harvard. He had worked in the Foreign Service under multiple presidents, at this time under Kennedy. He eventually became a deputy director under Shriver in starting the Peace Corps. He had served in the Foreign Service in many countries including Syria, India, and South Vietnam.

There was a story told that once Paul Geren and other Foreign Service officers were sitting around discussing where they would like to go next. The assignments would be made soon, and they knew that Paul Geren, with his experience, would get the assignment he wanted. One said France, another Switzerland, and around the group they went until they finally got to Paul Geren. The room was silent.

"I think," he said, "I would like to go to…"

Paul named a small country in the remote regions of Africa. One lady screamed.

"My God, Paul, you don't mean that!"

But Paul Geren did mean that. He had already been practicing on how to live without electricity and other creature comforts of our life. My meeting with him that evening was shortly before he was to leave. And he went.

Paul Geren is gone on now and is with the Lord, but it wasn't too long after Geren's death that I sat in that famous coffee house with Howard Rees and another young man. Rees, with his mischievous grin, kept referring to him as a "little Paul Geren." Here again, another generation, and Howard Rees had inspired a young man to begin moving into a calling and heading off to a small country in Africa. Trained as a businessman, the young man planned to help them understand some aspects of starting businesses.

It got to a point where once I picked up the *Washington Post* and saw that a major pastor in the D.C. area had resigned his pastorate and was going to become a counselor. The next time I was with Howard Rees I turned to him, "You met with that pastor, didn't you?"

"Yes," he said, "just before he made the decision."

WHAT IS GOD TELLING YOU TO DO?

My guess is that leaders across the city and beyond often came to Rees for advice. In his own quiet way, he asked them those questions about what God was telling them to do. It wasn't so much what Howard Rees and Paul Geren said that changed my life, but what they did. I found I wanted to be on the front line, feeling the tingle along with them of the coming Kingdom.

"Carl," Rees once told me, "I find I really can't trust someone unless they have been through an incredible amount of pain and suffering."

Thirty years later, I don't have a cane but walk with a limp, just like Howard Rees. I have the same mischievous grin, and I'm the one asking those questions of people. Like Rees, I often have a strange discernment in conversations with people about a pathway they should take. A copy of the Rembrandt *The Apostle Paul* is over my fireplace. I have a hard time trusting someone who hasn't suffered, who hasn't faced their wound. The mantle from those who mentor us often falls on us.

Dialog

1. Who are the active mentors in your life now?

2. Who are the past mentors in your life?

3. Who are the passive mentors in your life (from books and other materials)?

4. What men (if you are a man) or women (if you are a woman) in the movies do you most admire? Why?

5. What are the common aspects of these mentors or characters?

11

The Desire and Pursuit for the Kingdom of Heaven

*"Slowly they crawled up to the edge of the ring again, and peered through the cleft between the two jagged stones. The light was no longer bright, for the clear morning had faded...neither Frodo nor Merry could make out their shapes for certain; yet something told them that there, far below, were Black Riders assembling on the Road beyond the foot of the hill. 'Yes,' said Strider, whose keener sight left him in no doubt. '**The enemy is here!**'"*

—J. R. R. Tolkien, *The Lord of the Rings: The Fellowship of the Ring* [1], emphasis added

It is difficult to view the healings that Jesus did in terms of the mindset of the culture of the time as well as that of our culture. This is probably the most difficult chapter to follow, yet it carries some of the deepest truths.

THE CULTURAL MINDSET AT THE TIME OF JESUS

At the time of Jesus, all disease was thought to be the result of sin, or something that a person did or perhaps inherited from the sins of those who went before him or her. The demonic spirits binding the demoniac were viewed as the result of his sin. Leprosy, lameness, blindness—all were perceived as a result of sin of the person or the parents.

After Jesus healed the man by the pool of Bethesda, he told the man to "go and sin no more" (John 5:14). At another healing Jesus was asked who had sinned, him or his parents:

> *"Now as Jesus passed by, He saw a man who was blind from birth. And His disciples asked Him, saying, 'Rabbi, who sinned, this man or his parents, that he was born blind?' Jesus answered, 'Neither this man nor his parents sinned, but that the works of God should be revealed in him.'"*
>
> —John 9:1–3 NKJV

THE CONTEMPORARY MINDSET

Today, in our Western culture, disease is perceived as a result of germs or biological malfunctions. We have a very rational approach to healing, and it is difficult for us to accept any healing outside of this rational framework. When it does happen, at times, we might call it a miracle, but deep within we often feel there is some type of rational explanation that is simply beyond our understanding. For example, here are a few of the people who came to Jesus and were healed with our rational explanations of why they were ill:

Luke 13:10–17	Arthritis or spinal curvature
Luke 14:2	Dropsy
Mark 9:14–19	Epilepsy
Matthew 12:22	Deafness
Mark 4:39	Infection (Fever)

THE MINDSET OF JESUS

When God created the world and placed Man in it, He gave Man authority over the world and all that was in it. When Man fell to Satan, the world also fell, since God had given it to Man. Satan now had authority over both Man and the world. From Christ's perspective, disease is considered to be a consequence of the rule of the Enemy on earth. There was no illness or disease before the Fall, and no death.

With the Fall, disease and death entered the world. Jesus took authority over disease and, in doing so, established his Kingdom on earth and his reign in the hearts of those who would accept him. In the model prayer Jesus gave us, we pray, "may your kingdom be established, on earth as it already is in Heaven." Jesus, in healing, was birthing the Kingdom again on earth. This is very hard for us to understand in the West.

In many scriptures (Mark 5:23, 5:34, 5:56, 10:52) Ken Blue[2] points out that the Greek word *sozo*, is used, which translates as "to heal or make whole." The same word also means "to save." Jesus is treating the disease as if it belongs to a larger disease of evil. In the story of the paralyzed man who was let through the roof (Mark 2:1–12), Jesus makes it clear that he is not only physically healing the man, but saving him.

WHAT SHOULD OUR MINDSET BE?

The purpose of the healing is the birthing of the Kingdom of God and establishing it on earth today. Our mindset, like that of Jesus, is to see people well. We have authority, in his name, for physical, emotional, and spiritual healing. Jesus gives us that authority to do this in his name. Ken Blue tells several stories to illustrate this, of which this is one:

> *"A young man, who recently converted to Christ out of the occult, came to me for help when his hands became spastic. As he walked through my living room door, he held out his hands which resembled bird's claws. He was being medically tested for neurological disease, but he wanted prayer as well. I began to pray for him and almost immediately he sensed a spirit. I confronted it; it showed*

itself, and left. Within a few minutes, the young man's hands were back to normal and have remained so."[3]

ISSUES OF AUTHORITY AND OWNERSHIP

To understand the mystery of the relationship of prayer and healing, you must understand the history of God's authority and ownership. God created the earth and Man because he was and is love, and this perfect love requires an object (Man) and a deep sense of intimacy with Man. This is why God created Man and the world.

Talk to the top physicists today and they will tell you an interesting thing. If there was a Big Bang, it violated the Second Law of Thermodynamics.[4] In addition, the idea of Man was there in the first nanosecond of creation.[5] God had the idea of man before the creation of the world. With his foreknowledge, I believe he had the idea of *you* before the world was created!

> *"Oh yes, you shaped me first inside, then out;*
> *you formed me in my mother's womb.*
> *I thank you, High God—you're breathtaking!*
> *Body and soul, I am marvelously made!*
> *I worship in adoration—what a creation!*
> *You know me inside and out,*
> *you know every bone in my body;*
> *You know exactly how I was made,*
> *bit by bit, how I was sculpted from nothing into something.*
> *Like an open book, you watched me grow from conception to birth;*
> *all the stages of my life were spread before you,*
> *The days of my life all prepared before I'd even lived one day."*
>
> —Psalms 139:13–16 *The Message*

For this love to be real, God had to release to Man the choice of whether to love him or not. God also created the earth and gave Man the authority over the earth. It was Man who had the authority, given by God, to name the animals.

When Man fell to Satan, Man gave Satan authority on earth, as God had already released this authority to Man. The example mentioned earlier was that this is much like a landlord who lets you rent his apartment. The landlord still owns the apartment, but he releases authority to you and gives you the keys. You have the responsibility of proper stewardship of the apartment. If you fail to use the apartment properly, you are accountable to the landlord. In the same way, God still owns the earth and all that is in it:

> "The earth is the LORD's, and all its fullness,
> The world and those who dwell therein."
>
> —Ps. 24:1 NKJV.

God released the stewardship, or authority of the earth, to Man—who released it to Satan. The only way God could reclaim this authority and Man's relationship to him would be to become Man himself (Jesus) and reclaim the keys (authority) from Satan. This is exactly what God did. We live on a visited planet.

At the beginning of Jesus' ministry, Satan tempted Jesus. Satan tried a vicious attack on the identity of Jesus.

> "And the devil said to Him, 'All this authority I will give You, and their glory; for this has been delivered to me, and I give it to whomever I wish. Therefore, if You will worship before me, all will be Yours.'"
>
> —Luke 4:6–7 NKJV

Jesus refused him.

I like the way Mark tells the story of the ministry that follows. Mark is believed to have written his gospel from the sermons of Peter. It is from Mark, then, that we get a glimpse of Peter's impetuous personality. There is no vulnerable baby in Mark's gospel. There is only one sentence of introduction. Jesus literally explodes on the scene and we see the new Kingdom of Heaven crashing against the matrix of false reality built from our broken past. You see from the first chapter of Mark a constant litany of words like "immediately...", "at once...", "quickly...", and "without delay." It's as if Mark (or Peter) can't wait to tell the story.

By Mark 10:46 we see the incredible story of blind Bartimaeus telling Jesus (who asks what he wants), "I want to see!" Isn't that the cry of each of us? There is no washing of the eyes. Mark says he *immediately* received his sight. The first thing he sees is the face of Jesus. The Kingdom has come.

Elisha prays to open the eyes of his servant; Morpheus asks Neo if he wants to see. Paul writes to the Corinthians that he only sees dimly. Jesus weeps at the tomb of Lazarus because those with him could not see. Do you want to see?

In just a few years Jesus dies on a cross, descends to Hell, and takes the keys and authority back from Satan. On the third day, Jesus rises from the dead and soon stands before his followers, telling them **He** now has authority on *earth* as well as in Heaven:

> *"All authority is given to me on heaven and on earth..."*
>
> —Matt. 28:18

Then he ascended to Heaven, taking the keys with him. Sounds like the keys are lost now—but wait. He left with us the authority as long as we ask in his name...

> *"Most assuredly, I say to you, he who believes in Me, the works that I do he will do also; and greater works than these he will do, because I go to My Father. And whatever you ask in My name, that I will do, that the Father may be glorified in the Son. If you ask anything in My name, I will do it."*
>
> —John 14:12–14 NKJV

So there are now three kingdoms. The kingdom of Satan, the Kingdom of Heaven, and the kingdom of earth. We can claim the Kingdom of Heaven on earth if we ask in his name. As long as we have the intimacy with the Father and know the Father's agenda, we have authority to claim that agenda on earth. He has the keys!

> *"And I will give you the keys of the kingdom of heaven, and whatever you bind on earth will be bound in heaven, and whatever you loose on earth will be loosed in heaven."*
>
> —Matt 16:19 NKJV

> *"...and you have been given fullness in Christ, who is the head over every power and authority."*
>
> —Col 2:9–10 NIV

As we mentioned earlier, the word used for authority here is the Greek word *exousia*, which means ability, worker of miracles, strength. It's used in Luke 9:1 and again in Matt. 10:1 when Jesus sends the disciples out. It is used again in reference to Jesus in the Great Commission. Look at the Great Commission in the gospels and the words of Jesus just before His ascension. Jesus always had the power. Power was never an issue. Jesus regained the authority at the Cross. Jesus tells His followers that:

- He (Jesus) has all power (*dunamis*) and authority (*exousia*)

- He delegates this to his followers, giving them, in turn, this power and authority

- He sends them out in terms of this authority and power

- They are responsible (accountable) for following this command

ESTABLISHING A BEACHHEAD

Few people learning about the issue of prayer and its relationship to healing understand the dangers and power that are involved. In the name of Jesus you are taking authority and the power for the healing. *That is the last thing the Enemy wants.* The Enemy doesn't even want you to know that there is a war going on.

Salvation begins at the healing moment, but is imperfect. It is an ongoing process that begins at that moment. The war for our hearts continues. A good illustration here is the example of D-Day when the allied troops landed at Normandy. This established a beachhead from which the war was ultimately won on V-E Day, many battles later. The movie *Saving Private Ryan* shows some of the cost of that battle, with a few remaining solders looking at the dead and dying around them. Only a remnant was left, but that was enough. They had established a beachhead from which they could continue and win the war. A secular beachhead is a small geographic area that acts as a staging area for invading forces. *It is often secured at a high cost because of its strategic nature in the war.*

In the same way, in spiritual warfare there are often beachheads that must necessarily be secured at high cost to a city, church, or individual. Lives will be lost in the process because the war is real until Christ returns to complete the establishment of his Kingdom. Sometimes we might pray for someone and then see their healing begin. A beachhead has been established. A strategic place has been established for the coming of the Kingdom in that person's life and the lives of others that see this. But there are many battles for this person that are yet to come. We celebrate the establishing of the beachhead.

When Sandy was diagnosed with the leukemia, it was a late diagnosis. The doctors were afraid they would not be able to get the chemotherapy started in time to save her. After the first round, she was still alive, but the leukemia cells were back again. With this type of leukemia, we were told, they could only do two rounds of chemotherapy.

They did a second, and final, round. After the second round the white cell count dropped to zero again, but would not come back up. Sandy was without any immune system, and pneumonia was moving in rapidly. As a last resort they used a new genetic drug that had only been on the market a month to kick the white count. The white count came up immediately without the leukemia cells. Miracle two.

The doctors warned us, however, that with this type of leukemia there was a 90% chance the leukemia would be back within a year, and the cells that came back would be resistant to any type of chemotherapy. We were strongly advised to get the bone marrow transplant, which would increase survival chances to 50%.

The transplant went well, but a few weeks after the transplant Sandy (now an outpatient) suddenly went catatonic on us. An ambulance took her to the hospital again and doctors started around-the-clock testing to find the cause. Sandy came out of the catatonic state, but had severe mental problems with memory loss, unable to process what was going on around her, and extreme restlessness (hyperactive). After three weeks an MRI showed the source of the problem—multiple lesions in the brain. I called my pastor (Peter) and told him they were thinking of drilling holes in her skull to permit drainage. Peter said they would start fasting and praying. Another prayer warrior, Carol Bouschor, called me soon.

"I'm coming up," she said (a 3 ½ hour drive).

"She won't even recognize you," I said.

"You don't understand," Carol replied.

I prayed. The next morning Carol and I walked in Sandy's room at breakfast time and she was completely restored and normal, eating her breakfast. A neurologist was called in, and his testing showed nothing amiss. Another MRI was done a few days later and showed everything was completely normal. The lesions were gone. I got a copy of the final medical report. The report said it was "spontaneous remission." That's the way they spell "miracle."

So why did she die about nine months later when the transplant rejected her body? *There's a war going on. The Enemy is here.*

THE COMING OF THE KINGDOM

It seems that so little has been accomplished in this dark, dark world when we pray for healing of a single person and we see that happen. It's as though we now have a tiny shaft of light in this dark world. But as John says, the light shines in the darkness and the darkness can't put it out.

With revival breaking in Argentina, pastors have traveled there for years to see it first-hand. A friend told me he traveled to a prison there where only the most hardened of criminals are sent. Revival was sweeping the prison. As he entered the prison, one of the men approached him and told him quite bluntly, "We aren't in prison. You are."[6]

A young man in our church, Mark, traveled to Africa to minister there and came down with malaria in one of the remote villages. As Mark lay on a pallet with tremors and dying, a boy of about ten came in and prayed for him. Mark tells me the boy could hardly speak any English, and what English he did know was spoken in a very broken way. As the boy prayed, however, beautiful English words flowed from the boy's mouth that were certainly beyond the kid's knowledge. My friend was instantly healed. As Mark and the boy shared later, Mark realized the kid had very little rational knowledge about the world. He didn't know the earth revolved around the sun or what the stars were. The kid wasn't bound by rational knowledge and did what we would consider irrational. Another pastor from Africa visiting our church told me the story of his wife being raised from the dead.[7]

At some of these conferences I've met people that travel from one area to another where spiritual fires are breaking out, surfing what C. Peter Wagner calls the Third Wave of the Holy Spirit.

"Within it the sick are being healed, the lame are walking, demons are being cast out, and other New Testament manifestations of supernatural power are seen." [8]

The Kingdom of Heaven is coming, but it is always coming in tension with its counterpart until Jesus returns. When I take speakers out to lunch at these conferences, I hear stories you wouldn't believe if I told you.

In Mark 4 and Matthew 13 Jesus uses parables to try to explain the Kingdom of Heaven to us. The first is the parable of the sower. The seed of the Kingdom was all good seed, but it fell on a variety of soils. Some fell on hard ground and was snatched away by Satan. Some fell on shallow ground and can't develop roots—a failure of discipling. Others fell on thorny ground and were choked out by leisure, comfortable living, and the desire for power and wealth. Some seed fell on good ground, growing and producing until the harvest. All of the seed was good. The moral here is that sometimes the success of the Kingdom on earth can be snatched away by the Enemy.

In reading the other parables in this chapter, the same thread runs through all the parables. In the parables (as with the mustard seed and the yeast) you can see the significance of a few healings that may seem insignificant to us, but really are the trumpet sounds heralding the coming Kingdom. The lost coin (Luke 15:8), the pearl (Matt. 13:46), the treasure in the field (Matt. 13:44), and the parable of the talents (Matt. 24) were parables of the Kingdom.

RELEASING TO GOD'S AGENDA

One of the most difficult decisions in praying is often to be able to release ourselves to God's agenda. We can see the difficulty of this in the story of Lazarus, who was raised from the dead (John 11).

Jesus was ministering in the area where John had been baptizing when word came to him that Lazarus was sick. Mary was the one who had, earlier, poured perfume on the feet of Jesus. Mary, Martha, and Lazarus were all siblings. Jesus does not leave immediately, however, and remains where he is ministering for two more days. Then he tells his disciples they must go to Judea and Bethany, where Mary and Martha live. Judea would be a very dangerous area for Jesus to go to at this time, and the disciples reminded him. Jesus was determined to go. I like Thomas who says with deep resignation, "All right, let's go that we may die with him." So the disciples go with Jesus.

As Jesus arrives at Bethany, there is a large crowd of mourners. Lazarus has been in the tomb four days. He's dead. Really dead. Martha hears that Jesus is coming and leaves to meet him outside the town. She's pretty ticked off, saying that if He had come earlier Lazarus would not have died (her agenda). Notice, however, the faith of Martha in that she says God can do anything if it is done under the authority of Christ.

> *"Then Martha said to Jesus, 'Lord, if You had been here, my brother would not have died. But even now I know that whatever You ask of God, God will give You.'"*
>
> —John 11:21–22 NKJV

Notice there is no apparent worship from Martha at this point. Jesus is on his agenda, and reminds Martha here that it is never too late for his agenda. (As one of my mentors used to tell me, God's trains are always on time.) There are two important things here to note, however, and the faith issue is not the question. First, Martha has total trust in Christ's agenda. She submits herself to that agenda. Second, there is a brokenness in submitting to that agenda. Sometimes as children we submit to our parent's agenda, but do it grudgingly, griping all the time. You don't see that here. Martha submits willingly. Are we really willing to trust and submit when we pray, regardless of our personal desires?

When Martha returns, Mary gets up and with a large crowd goes out of the village to meet Jesus where Martha had met him. Mary falls on her knees and worships Jesus. Worship is essential in beginning our prayer. Mary is just as upset as Martha (and says so), but worships and, like Martha, submits to Jesus' agenda. They then, as a group, travel to the tomb of Lazarus.

As they stood at the tomb, the scripture says that Jesus wept. Why did he weep? Jesus already knew that Lazarus was alive again or would soon be. He knew the endgame. So why did he weep? He was weeping because of the unbelief in the crowd around him and because he knew Lazarus would eventually die again. Jesus then offers a prayer of thanksgiving to God, even though in human terms there is yet no sign that Lazarus is alive again. In the prayer Jesus gives the purpose for his delayed trip and the raising of Lazarus from the dead:

> "...that they may believe that you sent me."

The purpose was to show the coming of the Kingdom of God to a large crowd of witnesses. If he had come when they initially called him, only a small group would have seen the healing. Our agenda is often with Mary and Martha, we want our prayers answered quickly, take the healing, then get the show on the road again. Jesus here had the purpose of bringing the Kingdom of God to as many people as possible.

After the prayer Jesus calls in a loud voice, "Lazarus, come forth!"

Here's another issue that seems a paradox. Jesus could have emptied the entire cemetery if he had wished. My guess is that among those mourners there were some who had lost spouses, kids, and parents who were buried in that cemetery. He awakens only Lazarus, and then only for a time. Eventually, Lazarus will die again. The same is true in our healings. Death in this world is always inevitable unless Jesus comes back first. The key, again, is an authority issue. Jesus calls Lazarus *by name* to claim his authority over him and life and death.

Now read the story again, and ask yourself where you are in the story. There is a wide variety of attitudes here. Also be sure to read John 12:10 to see another attitude in the audience that was there.

Dialog

1. What evidence have you seen of the coming Kingdom in the last week?

2. What was the real temptation of Jesus at the beginning of his ministry in terms of authority and power?

3. Read John 14:12–14. How does this relate to your life?

4. Do you believe the miracles in the early church are still available to the Church today? Why or why not?

Notes

1. Unknown to the hobbits and the rest of the fellowship, Strider is really Aragon, the coming King. Within a few minutes "Strider" will have to initiate healing for Frodo, the hobbit, from a deadly attack of the enemy. Aragon's Kingship is not *really* revealed, however, until the final volume of the series, *The Return of the King*. Check the book: the wounding in this incident was to Frodo's left shoulder. The Black Riders were aiming for Frodo's heart. That is where the Enemy always tries to strike us. Frodo and the fellowship have yet to learn who Strider really is. How like the people of Nazareth that had trouble seeing the King among them. Or us.

2. Blue, Ken. *Authority to Heal.* (Intervarsity Press: Downers Grove, IL), 1987, p. 85–86

3. Ibid, p. 87

4. The Second Law of Thermodynamics, simply stated, says the universe is running down. The universe was once set to a high state of order (low entropy), and since then has been running down to the state of chaos from which is started (high entropy). The only way the universe could have been set to this high state of order is if

something came in from outside the system and did it. That is
exactly what Genesis says happened.

5. Glynn, Patrick. *God the Evidence: The Reconciliation of Faith and
    Reason in a Postsecular World.* (Prima Publishing: Rocklin, CA)
    1997

6. The prisoner was challenging my friend about his lack of authority
    in ministry and trying to live in a small story. In reality, my friend
    had suffered with chronic fatigue syndrome for years after he was
    in the Gulf War. He was suddenly healed, and remains healed,
    from the CFS with a single session with a well-known healer. He
    leads an incredible ministry today and has a lot of spiritual author-
    ity.

7. Townsend, Carl. *Catching the Wind: Finding Vision in a World of
    Chaos.* (available at http://www.netadventures.biz). 2000

8. Wagner, C. Peter. *The Third Wave of the Holy Spirit: Encountering
    the Power of Signs and Wonders.* (Vine Books: Ann Arbor). 1988, p.
    18

12

The Strategy for the Healing

*"People are the gatekeepers of change and healing. It is people who
have the visions and power, not the structures or the geographic
locations. The reason most visions fail is that the focus is on the
program, agenda, or the technology—rather than the people. God
trusts his visions to people."*

—Carl Townsend

Let's begin by defusing any brilliant hope you have when coming to
this chapter—perhaps the first chapter you are reading. There isn't any
strategy. Jesus always did it differently. We can, however, learn a few
things about healing from his ministry. There are some common ele-
ments in *all* of the healings and deliverances of Christ.

With the Church today there are healing traditions that vary with
cultures, denominations, and time. C. Peter Wager tells how when he
started his missionary work in Bolivia decades ago he chose to stay
away from the Pentecostals, as they had some pretty wild healing meet-
ings. He believed in the "germ theory" of diseases, whereas some of the
people in Bolivia he met thought diseases were caused by evil spirits.[1]
He and his team had injections, capsules, and rational medical knowledge. Only problem was, the Pentecostals were getting results. There
wasn't a lot of knowledge about the theological basis for what was
going on; but Wagner continued to study this. Under Don McGavran,
Wagner soon realized that the Church grows where the blind see, the
lame walk, the dead are raised, and other miraculous signs begin to
occur. Wagner made more trips to South America to study the phe-

nomenal and sudden growth of the Church there from this Pentecostal movement that he had once shunned.

From Wagner's state-side ministry, he soon met John Wimber, who had started a church in his living room that quickly grew to 6000. Wagner and Wimber were seeing the same miraculous signs in their own ministry. Their teamwork soon evolved to a class at Fuller Theological Seminary on this new wave of the Holy Spirit.[2] Today we are beginning to realize that God's healing is not bounded by our theology, rational science, or anything. After all, God's the boss. Medicines and our doctors are still very important, but we also need to deal with the underlying causes of disease. We don't need to judge others on how they do it or worry about theological judgments on how God uses us. We all share the common assumption that God wants us well and will heal the sick and deliver people from their demonic spirits.

We pray for change to take place in our lives, the church, or in the city. When occurs, it will not be from programs, structures, or organizations. It will be from people who are empowered and enabled by the Holy Spirit. God trust his visions to people, people committed to him and to the healing he wants to give the world. *People* are the gatekeepers of change and healing.

THE COMMON ASSUMPTIONS

There are common healing assumptions, however, that seem to be true with Christ and all traditions of the faith:

- Prayer

- Listening

- Compassion

- Risk-taking

And the healing, when it does come, is always a mystery.

Prayer and Healing

Jesus spent a lot of time praying and talking with his Father. When he did healing or deliverance, however, prayer did not seem to be an integral part of the healing. Instead, Jesus *spoke* the healing; that is, the power and authority was in the spoken word of Christ.

We see this even in Genesis, as God created the world from the *spoken word*. The creation versions begin "And God said…" and end with "and it was so."

When God and later Christ came into the chaos, they spoke the word with authority and power, and it happened. The same is true of the Holy Spirit today. The disciples tried some of this "speaking" during their time of ministry with Christ, but the Holy Spirit had not yet come and they only had the power that Christ had delegated to them.

After the death and resurrection of Christ, the Holy Spirit came at Pentecost. It was the Holy Spirit, acting through Peter and John that healed the lame man at the temple gate in Acts 3. Peter *spoke* the healing. This led to the birth of the Church, the powerful preaching ministry in the life of Peter, and the eventual conversion of Paul. And that was just the beginning! Prayer became an integral part of the healing process, for it was through prayer they received the mind of the Holy Spirit and could act from that. Today's Christian, like those in the book of Acts, receives the mind of the Holy Spirit through prayer and then acts from the same authority and power Christ had with only a spoken word.

The Greek word for this "word with power" is *rhema,* was mentioned earlier and is used in Eph. 6:7 to denote the only offensive weapon, in addition to prayer, that the Christian carries. It does not refer to the Bible as such (it didn't even exist at that time) but rather to a serendipity word (*paga* word), given by the Holy Spirit, that carries power (*dunamis*) and authority (*exousia*) as it is spoken.

The healer can use the *rhema* word to rebuke any demonic spirits and their control over the personalized evil. When Jesus healed Peter's mother-in-law, Jesus rebuked the demonic spirits when she apparently had what we would call an infection and fever (Luke 4:39). In Mark 9:25 we see Jesus rebuking the demonic spirits again in the healing of the boy with convulsions. See also Luke 4:36, Luke 9:42, and Matt. 17:18. He rebukes the storms in Matt. 8:26 and Mark 4:39.

There may be issues in the person who needs healing that will anger you, such as homosexuality, an abortion, poor moral values, lust…the list is endless. Your fight, however, is not against the person but the demonic forces that have gained authority. Love the person, fight and rebuke the demonic spirits.

Personal Praying for Healing

In the introduction two questions were mentioned that are critical to understanding the issue of healing. First, on the question of why didn't Sandy get well I was asking the wrong question. The question was not why Sandy didn't get well but what was God trying to do through her illness and death. That was not a question I wanted to face, but that's the one God forced me to face. My greatest fear was losing her, and now God was forcing me to understand his love by facing that fear. His love was greater than my fear.

The second question mentioned in the introduction is more complex but very important. In listing the prayer warriors I studied under, all but one on that list was a man. Why was that? The answer here was that the message I needed to hear had to come from a man. I had to hear that I had the strength for the adventure, the battle, and pursuit. That message can only come from another man. Never from a woman. The prayers of women were (and are) *very* important and protected me at many of those prayer conferences; but for my own healing I had to hear a specific message from a man that I had the strength for the adventure, battle, and pursuit. I also had to see the message demonstrated.

Listening

An important beginning step is to listen. If you are called as healer you must listen both to God and to the person who wishes to be healed. You can pray for God to speak, for you to hear, and pray for the ability to "hear" (both verbally and non-verbally) the other person.

An effective healer learns that his or her relationship with the Lord must be rich in intimacy and with a clear conscience if they are to hear the Lord. The heart must be clean before the Lord. Ask the Lord to reveal any unconfessed sins and repent of these. Acknowledge your total dependence on the Holy Spirit, and ask God to release any pre-conceived ideas and desires you have about the healing.

Remember the story of Moses at the foot of Mt. Sinai *demanding* God to reveal his plan? Pretty audacious, I would say. Yet later, in Numbers 14, Moses apparently now knows the plan and moves the hand of God to stay the destruction of the entire Israelite nation because they are essential to the plan. Nehemiah is able to claim God's help in the return of the Israelite nation and the rebuilding of the wall because he knew the plan. Esther knew the plan, and risked her life for it. In the same way, if your heart is true, God will reveal his plan and your part in making it happen.

In the same way, you must listen to the person who desires the healing. Don't try to give answers. Instead, ask questions. What is their desire? Where is the real healing needed? The person who desires the healing may have deep wounds from the past that are not even in the conscious level any more. Like the chains on the cover of this book, the binding is in the subconscious level. Like the chains, we see the bindings as distorted. We don't see them as they really are unless we ask God to reveal them. The person who is the healer has to be able to hear what the wounded person cannot tell him or her. The Holy Spirit can reveal this to the healer. You must also remember that about 90% of the communication is at the non-verbal level. The healer must learn to listen for these non-verbal clues.

An effective healer learns that the roots of many physical ailments (particularly chronic illnesses) are rooted in past emotional wounds. Sometimes the roots are far in the past, unconscious, and sometimes even cross-generational. Praying can often help in the discovery of this binding. Don't be too quick to just run with the latest event. You want to learn the pattern and why it repeats itself. Remember that *nothing* is hard-wired in the physical.

Just yesterday I went to get some blood drawn for a test. I was able to discern that the girl drawing the blood was angry about something. There were no verbal clues. She was pleasant, acting her job and doing everything right. I could have risked and asked why she was angry, but didn't take that risk. God told me later, however, that I could have simply told her what a wonderful day God had given us. She probably would have reacted, and then the door would be open. If we pray rightly, God will show us how to open the door. I'm still learning. This simple strategy shown here involves bringing praise into the situation to force a confrontation.

Compassion

The sense of compassion is there in all of the healings of Christ. Scripture after scripture shows that time and time again Christ is moved by the crowds, seeing them as sheep without a shepherd. He weeps at the tomb of Lazarus. There are times, as before he crosses the Sea of Galilee to the demoniac, that he seems to literally wear himself out trying to heal those in the crowds that came to him.

In its most prophetic form today, the healer takes on the suffering of the broken as if the brokenness and pain is his or her own and then prays into this for healing. This also takes the form of a mercy gift. This can be between two people as the pray-er takes on the pain of the person they are praying for. It can also, at times, involve praying for an entire people group and taking on the pain of that group.

The real prayer is always for the coming of the Holy Spirit and the Kingdom. When my wife was sick, as I prayed for her I took on her pain and suffering as if it was my own. This compassion becomes an active force, or *dunamis*, in the healing process. I knew, from research that has been done on stress that with the loss of my wife there would be about a 90% probability of my body taking on a major disease in the next year from this particular type of stress. From this knowledge, I was able to put down strategies and prayers to deal with it. One component, for example, was the purchase of a very good keyboard for playing hours and hours of music. The only illness I faced during that time was shingles, and it was miraculously cured in less than a week. If the intimacy with God is there, this compassion is not a choice. It is just there.

Healing prayers can, and should, be lifted for entire people groups where there is wounding. John Dawson, for example, has done much in leading our nation in identificational repentance.[3] In this example Christians have identified with the wounds of the Native Americans. Even though this initial wounding occurred generations ago by people who are no longer alive, the curse that has traveled through time can be broken by identifying with those wounded, asking forgiveness, and then taking risks that complete the healing process. In the same way, Bob Beckett has led in identificational repentance in Hemet, California and in so doing has seen a dramatic amount of healing in that city.[4]

Risk-Taking

Do you know how to train an elephant so he doesn't wander off? Off in those remote countries they tie a rope to one of his legs and then to a tree. The elephant can only wander away from the tree to the length of the rope. Finally after some time, the trainer removes the rope. The elephant still doesn't wander too far from the tree.

Bound by our own lack of faith and our comfortable life, we are culturally trained not to wander too far from the tree. As men, we lose the manhood that God gave us. We lose the woman because we have lost our manhood. We no longer take risks. We want to see, but we dare not open our eyes. Like the servant of Elisha, we don't see what God has provided for us in the battle. We need the Elisha's in the church to pray our eyes will be open. There is a war going on, and most of us don't know it or see it.

The healer is always taking risks. Whether he's asking a guy in a wheelchair to stand up, asking someone why they are angry or asking a broken lady about her relationship with her father, the healing involves taking risks. You may claim authority in the name of Christ over one demonic spirit, only to find a dozen more are suddenly all stirred up. That's what it's all about. You are on the brink of a disaster and the brink of a miracle at the same time.

As a result, you might hang back because you don't trust what God is telling you, or you may move forward and take the risk. Secular war is the same way. You don't have all the information. Do you act on intuition and the pieces of information you have, or do you wait for more information? Spiritual warfare can be a lot like that.

Yet if you don't take the risks, the Kingdom will never come. It's always a leap of faith, and there is always a mystery.

WHEN GOD SAYS NO

God always answers our prayers, but sometimes he says no. David wanted to build a new Temple, God said no.

Another problem is that God may be answering our prayers, but the warfare level is so high the answer is delayed. You think he said no, but we must simply persevere with the prayer on our end. You can see this in Daniel 10. God answered Daniel's prayer, but it took three weeks. Read why in Daniel 10:12. After three weeks this guy appears with a description that looks like Christ himself. He gives two reasons the prayer *was* answered: Daniel sought to gain understanding and he humbled himself. The answer was delayed, however, because a fierce battle in the heavenlies that lasted twenty-one days and involved some kind of territorial guy. Michael, one of the angels, eventually came to help him.

We tend to define healing on our own terms. God defines it in terms of the coming Kingdom. When you sit weeping because you see yourself losing the battle, God is weeping as well.

One issue that often is difficult is deciding when to let a vision go and when to fight for it. When I was paralyzed, I fought, and fought hard, to walk again although the doctors said it would be impossible. (Actually, I never heard the doctors say I wouldn't walk. Even hearing it would have risked my taking ownership on the statement. My wife told me later what the doctor had said as he stood by my bed.) When my wife was dying she tried to hold on to a vision of healing as I had; but in doing that we were not able to process the feelings about death and leaving each other for awhile. It boils down to the difference between hope and faith.

Here's the way I explain the difference. My cat is snoozing. Suppose I get up and head in the general direction of his food dish. If the cat jumps up and runs to the dish, tripping me up, even though I'm not going to the dish—that's faith. If he stays there, cocks his ear, and waits to hear if the can opener runs, that's hope.

THE ROLE OF PRAISE

Praise is an integral part of the healing experience.

- Praise God before you begin the healing for what God is going to do. Notice that when Jesus was raising Lazarus from the dead, Jesus was praising God before there was any visible sign of Lazarus being alive again.

- Praise God during the healing experience. Satan doesn't like praise, and this keeps the Enemy away.

- Finally, praise God when you end the experience. Sometimes there may appear to be no change (as with Jesus and Lazarus after the prayer), but you have set in motion certain forces. You will know and begin to feel those forces are starting to change things. Praise God for what is happening.

This issue of praise is so important I keep a music keyboard near my computer—a very good keyboard. It's not connected to the computer at the moment, but often (not once, many times) I can repair the computer by playing the keyboard. It's not so much that the keyboard music changes the computer, but it changes me. I then have the authority and power to fix the computer. The same idea also works when I'm praying for people, as people are much more valuable to the Lord than the computer.

Even as I write this today, I periodically stop to play a praise CD. My favorite at the moment is *Revival in Belfast*, and I've played Robin Mark's "Days of Elijah" on this several times today.

Dialog

1. What do you think about the statement: There really is no strategy that Jesus used in healing?

2. Who can you lift up in prayer for healing? What are your expectations?

3. What risks have you taken in healing prayer this week?

4. What does you church believe about healing? Does it need to be changed? How can you change it?

Notes

1. Wagner, C. Peter. *The Third Wave of the Holy Spirit: Encountering the Power of Signs and Wonders.* (Vine Books: Ann Arbor). 1988, p. 21–22

2. _____, *Signs and Wonders Today: The Remarkable Story of the Experimental Course MC510-Signs, Wonders, and*

Church Growth at Fuller Theological Seminary. (Christian Life Magazine, 396 E. St. Charles Rd., Wheaton, IL 60187). 1983

3. Dawson, John. *Healing America's Wounds.* (Regal: Ventura, CA). 1994

4. Beckett, Bob. *Commitment to Conquer.* (Chosen Books: Grand Rapids). 1997 (See also the Transformations I tape.)

13

The Role of the Church in Healing

"At the center of all this, Christ rules the church. The church, you see, is not peripheral to the world; the world is peripheral to the church. The church is Christ's body, by which he speaks and acts, by which he fills everything with His presence."

—Eph. 1:22 *The Message*

"The Church in the West today presents too easy a target for Satan. We do not believe we are at war. We do not know where the battleground is located, and, in spite of our weapons, they are neither loaded nor aimed at the right target. We are unaware of how vulnerable we are. We are better fitted for a parade than an amphibious landing."

—Ed Silvoso[1]

"The Church, as the Body of Christ, has the business of liberating the captives, recovering the sight of the blind, enabling the lame to walk, bringing the good news to the poor, and (yes) raising the dead."

Jesus spent almost all of His life either doing healing and deliverance, teaching, or talking with his Father. When Jesus ascended back to the Father, he left that charge to his followers, who would be guided by the Holy Spirit. Jesus was telling us that we, as the Church, as the Body of Christ, now have the role of taking on his mission, guided by the Holy Spirit. There is no way the Church can escape that mandate. If the Church isn't doing it, it has failed its mission. It's that simple.

WHAT IS THE CHURCH?

The Greek word used in the New Testament to describe the church was *ekklesia*, which means the called out, or a gathering of the called out. The next question, quite simply, would be from what are we called and to what are we called?

We've already discussed much of the "from what." We are called out of the chaos, the brokenness, the Decapolis, the illusion of the Matrix, the purposeless life.

To answer the "to what" is more difficult. How can a person understand if they have never seen it? We are called to adventure, a battle, a pursuit at a level we could never understand. Not even Neo (in *The Matrix*) could see it until he had taken the red pill. We are called to a purpose and an identity that are unique. We are called to love and be loved in a romance so intense that we are captured by this and want to stay there forever, and we will. We are called to peace, to place, to freedom, to hope, to duty, to sanctification, to grace. The word used for "call" in the New Testament is *kalein*, which was used in asking someone to a banquet or feast.

The mission is a bold one. Not only are we called to the healing of the individual, but also to the healing of the city, the nation, and finally the world. We go not in our own authority, but in the name of Jesus.

No one person could do this alone. This is why the Church, as the fellowship of the believers, is so important. The Church is the very Body of Christ, with all of the authority and power Christ had when he walked this earth.

I wonder what Christ thought when he looked at his early disciples and realized it was this motley gang that was going to have to carry on everything he was doing after he was gone. Sure, they tried it when he was around and generally ended up blowing it. *He wanted them to feel the helplessness of them trying to do it on their own.* Finally, he told them just to wait for the Holy Spirit and then Jesus checked out. And they did wait. When the Holy Spirit came, it changed everything. Now they had authority and power that Christ gave them with the Holy Spirit. Now they were actually dangerous to any established order. The people most threatened by this new church were the religious leaders themselves.

In the movie *Chocolat*, we see Vianne (Juliette Binoche) with her daughter arriving at a remote French village and opening a small chocolate shop. Vianne has spent her life wandering and has no "place." The local church sees the shop as sensuous, sinful, and (horrors) even open during Lent. Sermons are preached against her audacity. As others enter the story, they also have no place. The mayor's wife has left him, and he seems lost and lonely without any purpose other than to close the little chocolate shop. The grandmother (Judi Dench) is estranged from her daughter (Carrie-Anne Moss) and grandson. Roux (Johnny Depp), a river boat wanderer, is another one without place. The village church is powerless. There is no forgiveness, redemption, celebration, or healing. You have a village of wounded people.

In Vianne's little chocolate shop, however, the chocolate becomes a symbol of the free Grace that God gives. Vianne gives away her chocolates to those in need. The shop soon becomes church—a place where bonds are broken, forgiveness and repentance occurs, reconciliation and healing takes place, and there is celebration. At the same time, nothing is happening at the established "church." The little shop is an enigma, but people are choosing to be a part of what is happening there. By the end of the movie, it is Easter and the entire village is transformed (re-birthed) and healed and the people are dancing in the street. Vianne is looking to the future wanting to meet more needs and willing to fight the battles to see that happen. The people in the little chocolate shop became church, breathing life into the community and restoring the established church.

Frodo, in *Lord of the Rings*, is not capable on his own of completing his mission and saving Middle Earth. It takes the Fellowship of the Ring to complete the mission, with each of these in the fellowship doing what they were supposed to do and risking everything. In *The Matrix*, Neo can't destroy the Matrix alone. Morpheus, Trinity, and a few others face the challenge of the mission with him, sometimes putting their own lives on the line.

I have met people in my journey who think they can do this on their own. I have met churches that think they can transform the city on their own. It doesn't work that way. When Jesus prayed for us in the Garden, look how he prayed.

> *"I do not pray for these alone, but also for those who will believe in Me through their word; that they all may be **one**, as You, Father, are in Me, and I in You; that they also may be **one** in Us, **that the world may believe that You sent Me**. And the glory which You gave Me I have given them, that they may be **one** just as We are **one**: I in them, and You in Me; that they may be made perfect in **one**, and **that the world may know that You have sent Me**, and have loved them as You have loved Me."*

—John 17:20–24 NKJV, emphasis added

Later the Apostle Paul, writing to the church at Ephesus, encourages unity before speaking of the Gifts of the Spirit.

> *"I, therefore, the prisoner of the Lord, beseech you to walk worthy of the calling with which you were called, with all lowliness and gentleness, with longsuffering, bearing with one another in love, endeavoring to keep the **unity** of the Spirit in the bond of peace. There is **one** body and one Spirit, just as you were called in **one** hope of your calling; **one** Lord, **one** faith, one baptism; **one** God and Father of all, who is above all, and through all, and in you all."*

—Eph. 4:1–6 NKJV, emphasis added

Notice the repetition of the word "one" and "unity" in these passages. Notice the purpose of this unity—that the world may know that God has sent Jesus. You can't have unity without there being more than one person there. There is no such thing as the independent Christian, as the witness is from the unity.

THE WITNESS FROM THE UNITY

During the sixties I had the opportunity of working at the Potter's House coffeehouse in Washington, D.C.. This is a coffeehouse sponsored by the Church of the Saviour. It is run as a ministry (you don't make money there), but people visit there from all over the world.

On a typical work night, people would come in from all walks of life. Dates would stop in for pie and coffee. People from other countries would stop by who had read about it in a book somewhere. People hurting and lonely would stop by, often just wanting someone with whom to talk. While working there, I had to learn to identify those who were hurting and needed my ministry and distinguish them from others just looking for a relaxing time with their dates. I had to learn to listen, both verbally and non-verbally.

Our instructions for working there were quite simple. If someone came in and was hurting or needed healing and we had to choose between ministering to that person or ministering to someone hurting in our staff that night, we were to choose to minister to the staff person first. The focus was always on the unity.

At first this seemed strange. The person on the staff from our church would be there all evening. I also had their phone number and address and could reach them any time during the week. The person coming in the door was probably a stranger and may never return. After working there for awhile, however, I began to understand the reason. The unity we had between us was really the *only* witness we had. People would sense our unity when they came in and would come back again and again until they would literally beg us to tell them what was different there. I know, because earlier I had been the lonely, wounded, and depressed guy coming in. I would beg them to tell me stories about what God was doing there. And they would. And I came again and again until I wanted to stay there. I had found *paga*.

This unity issue is very, very important in the church. It is important not only in the local church, but in all the churches in a neighborhood and in a city. The task before the Church is too large for any one church and won't be accomplished unless the churches are working together. In most cases the Enemy's main strategy is to create disunity, a sense of pride, and to make one church think they have responsibility for transforming an entire city.

Ted Haggard, a pastor of a very large church in Colorado Springs, gives a great illustration of this in his book *Primary Purpose: Making It Hard for People to Go to Hell From Your City.* [1] If ten percent of his city of 300,000 attends any life-giving church and he wants his church to raise that to fifteen percent in a year, this means fifteen thousand new converts would have to be absorbed by his church. He doesn't have the facilities for this, much less the leadership for discipling and getting these new converts ministering in terms of their gifts. If, instead, he would be able to get two hundred churches healing and restoring 75 people in the year, the goal becomes quite manageable. As a result, he sees that his church with all of its resources should be helping the small churches in the city to do what God is calling them to do.

At least one church in Portland has taken Ted's message to heart. It's a large church, and they pay the pastor of an inner city church to stay in the inner city and minister there with his church. My personal experience, though, is that in Portland and other cities it is hard to get pastors working together strategically to accomplish transformational goals that can really change the city economically, socially, politically, and spiritually. That's not going to be done without the Holy Spirit and the release of the churches to the Holy Spirit. Wherever this has happened (and it has) it was because the city church had one prayer—the visitation of the Holy Spirit. And this prayer was made in unity.

THE BIG VISION STATEMENT

Now let's go back to the big vision statement of Jesus we mentioned earlier. The vision statement is in Matt. 11:4–5 in the reply of Jesus to John's messengers and also in Luke 4:18–21. In John 14:12–14 Jesus says that those who believe in him will be able to do these same mighty works and more that the Father may be glorified. Let's look at it again:

> *"The person who trusts me will not only do what I'm doing but even greater things, because I, on my way to the Father, am giving you the same work to do that I've been doing. You can count on it. From now on, whatever your request along the lines of who I am and what I am doing, I'll do it. That's how the Father will be seen for who he is in the Son. I mean it. Whatever your request in my name, I'll do."*
>
> —John 14:12–14 *The Message*

The beginning of this fulfillment is seen in Acts 3 with the healing of the lame man and the birth of the Church. I not only believe this same power is available today; but I also have seen it.

Just as individuals are given certain spiritual gifts, individual churches are given specific giftings. Just as individuals must work together in a local church with their gifts, just so churches must work together with their giftings to transform a city. To quote Christ, both as individuals and as churches we are salt and light.

Regardless of the strategy, the process brings change and those involved in leading the change are an enigma to the rest of the culture. Even with the healings that are brought by the change, however, people feel threatened. Look at the threatened religious leaders at the healing of the lame man in Acts 3.

THE STRATEGY

Again, as with the individual, there is no real "strategy," as such, for the healing of the church. I've watched the transformation videos from the Sentinel Group, and a great dialog process after watching these is to try to define what were the common factors in all the city and regional healings. What enabled the church and the city to be healed? Each story is radically different. To really explore what was in common you need to read *Informed Intercession* by George Otis, Jr.. Otis says that he found five factors for these transformed and healed communities:

1. Persevering leadership

2. Fervent, united prayer

3. Social reconciliation

4. Public power encounters

5. Diagnostic research and spiritual mapping

Although each of these seem to occur again and again with the healed communities, the first two were common to *all* of the transformed and healed cities. In most cases, the entire healing process of a city or region was initiated from one or two people who persevered in leadership and intercessory prayer saying, as with John Knox, "Give me Scotland lest I die." Are you willing to say this about your church? Your city?

The second factor in *all* of these healings was the fervent, united prayer. In some of these stories people prayed for weeks, months, and whatever it took until God visited them and the healing took place. There was no healing, however, unless the prayer was there. The prayer was not so much for healing, but a petitioning for the coming of the Holy Spirit.

More often today, I think, we see the coming of the Kingdom in our cities much like a dream my former pastor had.

> *"Little pieces of something like burning sagebrush blowing in the wind as little fires across a parched desert. Sometimes they bump into each other and together they burn brighter and stronger. They then blow on across the desert."*

Where the churches burn like this, they draw the hurting and wounded much like a flame draws moths. There is so much brokenness in today's world, and few churches meet this at the level where it needs to be met—the heart. In the early days of my church, we were drawing almost all of our congregation from the wounded and rejects from other churches. The church grew so fast we had to go to two services. This didn't solve the problem, as everybody came to both services because they were afraid they would miss something.

With the wars of time, we are a smaller church now, but the remnant that remains contains people with wonderful giftings, deep hearts, and committed to intercessory prayer. We still attract the wounded, and if you visited you would hear incredible testimonies. My church is much like I was at the beginning of this story: we know we need to be committed to learning more about prayer and praying.

Dialog

1. Describe your vision of what a church should really be like.

2. Do you know any church like this?

3. How is it different from other churches you know about?

4. If you are in a particular church, why are you at this particular church?

5. Can a parachurch organization be a church? Why or why not?

Notes

1. Silvoso, Ed. *That None Should Perish: How to Reach Entire Cities for Christ Through Prayer Evangelism.* (Regal: Ventura, CA). Unknown copyright date.

2. Haggard, Ted. *Primary Purpose: Making it Hard for People to Go to Hell From Your City.* (Creation House: Orlando, FL). 1995

APPENDIX

Selected Healings of Jesus

Date (A.D.)	Healing	Location	Matthew	Mark	Luke	John
27	Mass healing (all implied)		4:23-24			
	Samaritan woman at the well	Samaria				4:5-42
	Healing of Nobleman's son	Cana				4:46-54
	Rejection at Nazareth	Nazareth			4:16-30	
	Demoniac healed on Sunday	Capernaum		1:21-28	4:31-37	
	Mass healing	Capernaum	8:16-17			
	Peter's mother-in-law, others	Capernaum	8:14-17	1:29-34	4:38-41	
	Leper healed	Galilee	8:1-4	1:40-45	5:12-16	
	All healed				5:15-16	
	Paralytic healed	Capernaum	9:1-8	2:1-12	5:17-26	

Date	Healing	Location	Matthew	Mark	Luke	John
(A.D.)						
	Mass healing (all implied)		9:35			
	Heals lame man	Jerusalem				5:1-47
	Withered hand healed	Galilee	12:9-14	3:1-7	6:6-11	
	Multitudes healed	Sea of Galilee	12:15-21	3:7-12	6:17-19	
	Centurion's servant healed	Capernaum	8:5-13		7:1-10	
	Raises widow's son from the dead	Nain			7:11-17	
	Sinful woman forgiven				7:36-50	
28	Gadarene Demoniac	Decapolis	8:28-34	5:1-20	8:26-27	
	Jairus' daughter raised from the dead		9:18-26	5:21-43	8:40-56	
	Woman with hemorrhage healed		9:20-22	5:25-34	8:43-48	
	Two blind men have sight restored		9:27-31			

Date	Healing	Location	Matthew	Mark	Luke	John
(A.D.)						
	Multitude healed				9:11	
	Mute demoniac healed		9:32-35		11:14-15	
	Multitude healed (all implied)		9:35			
	Blind, mute demoniac healed		12:22-24			
	Nazareth rejects Christ again		13:53-58	6:1-6		
29	Sick of Gennesaret healed	Gennesaret	14:34-36	6:53-56		
	Phoenician woman healed	Phoenicia	15:21-28	7:24-30		
	Afflicted healed	Decapolis	15:29-31			
	Deaf/mute healed	Decapolis		7:31-37		
	Blind man healed			8:13-26		
	Epileptic boy healed		17:14-21	9:14-19	9:37-43a	
	Forgives adulteress	Jerusalem				7:53-8:11
	Man born blind healed					9:1-41

Date	Healing	Location	Matthew	Mark	Luke	John
(A.D.)						
	Crippled woman healed				13:10-17	
	Healing of man with dropsy	Perea			14:1-24	
	Raising of Lazarus	Bethany				11:1-46
30	Heals ten lepers				17:12-19	
	Blind Bartimaeus healed	Jericho	20:29-34	10:46-52	18:35-43	
	Ten lepers healed				17:11-19	
	Zacchaeus healed	Jericho			19:1-10	
	Anointing of Mary	Bethany	26:6-13	14:3-9		12:2-8
	Healing of soldier's ear	Gethsemane			22:51	

0-595-29308-5